Karol Fireman
Cristiane A.Nascimento
Francisca M.N. da Silva

Exposure of tobacco farmers to pesticides

Karol Fireman
Cristiane A.Nascimento
Francisca M.N. da Silva

Exposure of tobacco farmers to pesticides

Biochemical and haematological profile

ScienciaScripts

Imprint

Cover image: www.ingimage.com

This book is a translation from the original published under ISBN 978-613-9-63822-2.

Publisher:
Sciencia Scripts
is a trademark of
Dodo Books Indian Ocean Ltd. and OmniScriptum S.R.L publishing group

120 High Road, East Finchley, London, N2 9ED, United Kingdom
Str. Armeneasca 28/1, office 1, Chisinau MD-2012, Republic of Moldova, Europe
Printed at: see last page
ISBN: 978-620-7-70368-5

PRESENTATION

This book is the result of a partnership between the Arapiraca Campus of the Federal University of Alagoas (UFAL), the Reference Centre for Workers' Health (CEREST) in Arapiraca (AL) and the National School of Public Health of the Osvaldo Cruz Institute Foundation (ENSP / FIOCRUZ), led by professionals from these institutions from a multi- and inter-professional perspective.

The use of pesticides and the handling of crops such as tobacco has been a constant public health problem in Brazil and around the world. In regions where family farming is most affected by the consequences of pesticides, characterising the blood count and serum biochemical profile of individuals exposed to pesticides in tobacco farming has become a necessity.

Interestingly, many authors have discussed the subject of pesticides and tobacco handling, but few studies have taken a similar approach to the one presented here.

This study therefore set out to analyse the profile of exposure to pesticides, the profile of serum biochemical test results from blood samples taken during the period of exposure, as well as the blood count in blood samples taken during the period of exposure, and to assess possible changes in biological variables between different subgroups of individuals. Offering health professionals a clinical and laboratory assessment of workers' health.

I believe that this book can take a fresh look at assessing the health of rural workers through routine examinations and deepen this discussion, which is so scarce in the literature.

SUMMARY

Brazil has become the largest consumer of pesticides in the world, accounting for 86% of these products in the Latin American market. Tobacco is one of the crops that uses pesticides on a large scale to increase its quality and productivity, and the municipality of Arapiraca is one of the main producers in Brazil. Exposure to pesticides without the necessary care and over the long term can cause acute or chronic poisoning, triggering a series of illnesses. In this respect, the identification of biomarkers that may indicate a potential physiological impairment of the organism and preventive measures are extremely important for the health of rural workers exposed to these substances. The aim of this study was to characterise the blood count and serum biochemical profile of tobacco farmers in order to identify variations that could be associated with exposure to pesticides. This is a cross-sectional analytical study in which 166 individuals took part in the biochemical and haematological assessment and answered a semi-structured questionnaire on sociodemographic data, lifestyle habits and occupational profile. A battery of haematological tests was carried out and the average values were compared between subgroups of individuals characterised by their exposure profile to the main chemical groups used. The characterisation of the study population shows that 60% were men, with an average age of 42, 62% had not completed primary school, a third of the sample were smokers, consuming an average of 12 cigarettes a day, 61% were alcoholics and of these 36.8% drank alcohol up to three times a week. Half of them called themselves mestizo and a third black and 79% of the farmers reported having direct contact with pesticides. The most commonly used pesticides were those belonging to the pyrethroid, neonicotinoid, strobilurin and organophosphate groups. The most frequently reported symptoms were nausea (70%), vomiting (42%) and vertigo (40%), with 83.9% of the individuals exposed to organophosphates showing muscarinic symptoms. The comparative analysis of the tests between different exposure subgroups showed significant differences for a number of variables. Individuals exposed to strobilurins had higher lactate dehydrogenase and gamma glutamyl transferase than those not exposed. Those exposed to organophosphates exhibited significantly different high-density lipoprotein and lipase than those not exposed. Women exposed to neonicotinoids had significantly higher red blood cells ($p = 0.035$), platelets ($p = 0.009$) and globulins ($p = 0.041$) than those not exposed. As for those exposed to pyrethroids, the women had significant haematocrit ($p=0.007$), haemoglobin ($p=0.009$) and phosphorus ($p=0.001$) compared to those not exposed. There were altered tests in the organophosphate groups (HDL, lipase and platelets), pyrethroids (potassium, haematocrit, haemoglobin, red blood cells, urea, ALT, phosphorus and uric acid), neonicotinoids (red blood cells, platelets, globulins, magnesium and urea) and strobilurins (LDH, GGT, lymphocytes, globulins and magnesium).In this study, we found that exposure to specific groups of pesticides induced significant differences in various serum biochemical parameters and in the blood count, suggesting that these pesticides interfere with the physiology of the individuals.

Keywords: Agrotoxics. Smoke farming. Biomarkers.

SUMMARY

CHAPTER 1

INTRODUCTION

Brazil is the largest exporter of tobacco in the world. Of all the agricultural products it produces, tobacco has been one of the main products on the export agenda (ASSOCIAÇÃO DOS FUMICULTORES BRASILEIROS, 2008). Among the factors that have driven this growth are the low costs of domestic production due to cheap labour involving the tobacco growers' families, and the fact that mechanisation is not necessary for cultivation. Situational factors such as the reduction in world stocks and tobacco production also favour the growth of this sector (FOOD AND AGRICULTURE ORGANISATION, 2003).

The tobacco industry, with its transnational companies such as Souza Cruz, has encouraged countries and farmers to grow tobacco in order to serve the market and make ever greater profits. The profits are remitted to the United Kingdom and the United States of America, outside the countries of production (CAMPAIGNING FOR TABACCO FREE KIDS, 2001).

In Brazil, tobacco production is concentrated in the South and Northeast. In the South, all the states are tobacco producers and economically dependent on private companies such as Universal Leaf Corporation and Souza Cruz. These have provided predictability and economic security for these growers. By commercialising and financing inputs for tobacco growing, these private companies have strengthened their ties with producers in Rio Grande do Sul (ALMEIDA, 2005).

Tobacco growing is a traditional activity in the north-east of Brazil and is found mainly in Bahia, Sergipe and Alagoas. It has established itself as one of the most important crops in the region since the beginning of colonisation (NADIR, 2004).

In Alagoas, the tobacco-growing region is concentrated in Arapiraca (Figure 1). This municipality is one of the most important in the state of Alagoas. As it is located in the heart of the agreste region of Alagoas, it serves the needs of the region as a commercial hub and historically its main source of income has been the commercialisation of tobacco (OLIVEIRA-SILVA et al., 2002).

The state of Alagoas was organised into macro- and micro-regions, in accordance with Normative IN GM/MS No. 2, of 6/4/2001, established by the Operational Standard for Health Care (NORMA OPERACIONAL DA ASSISTÊNCIA À SAÚDE /SISTEMA ÚNICO DE SAÚDE 01/01), approved by Ministerial Order No. 25, of 26 January 2001. Through this grouping, Arapiraca belongs to the 4th health macro-region of Alagoas with 24 municipalities and 615,650 inhabitants (20.2%) (ALAGOAS, 2002).

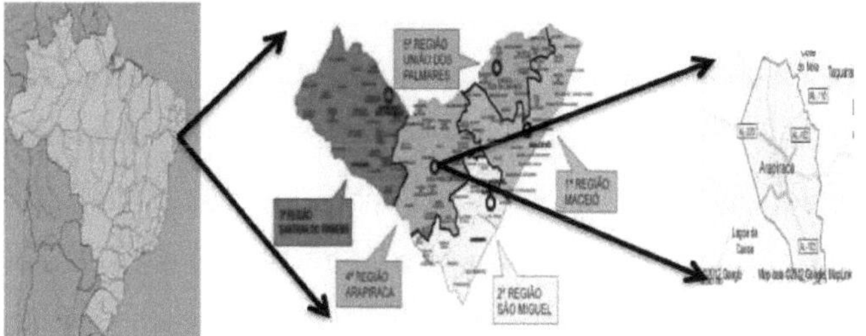

Figure 1 - Location of the municipality of Arapiraca, belonging to the 4ª health macro-region of Alagoas, 2007

Source. PDR-AL, 2002/IBGE, 2007. Alagoas, 2002.

In the city of Arapiraca, tobacco is mainly grown as "rope tobacco" and dark tobacco used to make cigars and cigarillos (NADIR, 2004). Production is concentrated on small family farms of up to 5 ha (MESQUITA, 2003). It requires intensive use of pesticides throughout the production cycle, a situation that can damage the health of the workers directly involved and also affects their families (CAVALCANTE, 2011) and harms the environment.

The development of this research is the result of actions initiated in the project entitled "The use of pesticides in northeastern Brazil and its impacts on the environment and human health", which is national in scope and funded by CNPq (MCT-CNPq/MS-SCTIE-DECIT/CT- Saúde - N° 24/2006). The macro-project was conducted by researchers from the National School of Public Health (ENSP/Fiocruz), who sought to promote an integrated assessment of the impact of pesticide use on the environment and human health in the north-eastern region of Brazil, emphasising tobacco cultivation in this region.

The study in Alagoas was divided into phases, the first between 2008 and 2010 with the study on "Evaluation of the working conditions of tobacco farmers in the municipality of Arapiraca (AL): contributions to the study on the perception of risk in rural workers exposed to pesticides", the second between 2009 and 2011 when the "Occupational profile and exposure to pesticides and nicotine of workers in the rural area of Arapiraca (AL) involved in tobacco cultivation" was identified and the third phase was carried out with the present study.

Pesticides have been associated with various adverse effects, in addition to poisoning. Bhatt et al. (1999) found that exposure to pesticides may be associated with an increased risk of developing neurodegenerative pathologies, especially Parkinson's disease. Immunological, haematological and endocrine effects have also been associated (RITZ & YU, 2000). Periodic exposure at low levels is known to produce a diversity of biochemical and cellular variations, some of which may be responsible for harmful biological effects reported in humans and rats (HERNÁNDEZ et al., 2005).

The lack of worker health monitoring programmes by health services makes it difficult to provide the necessary guidance and conduct to prevent diseases related to handling pesticides. The purpose of this study was therefore to examine the possible influence of pesticides on haematological and serum biochemical patterns in rural tobacco workers in the municipality of Arapiraca (AL), contributing to investigations into the health-disease process in this population.

CHAPTER 2

OBJECTIVES

2.1 General Objective

To characterise the blood count and serum biochemical profile of individuals exposed to pesticides in tobacco growing.

2.2 Specific Objectives:

- To identify the profile of exposure to pesticides using a semi-structured questionnaire;
- Carry out serum biochemical tests of relevant physiological variables on blood samples taken during the exposure period;
- Perform a haemogram on blood samples taken during the exposure period;
- To assess possible changes in the biological variables analysed between different subgroups of individuals, characterised by their exposure profile.

CHAPTER 3

LITERATURE REVIEW

3.1 Smoking

Tobacco growing in Brazil dates back to its discovery. Cultivated by the Indians, tobacco was sacred to them and was used in tribal ceremonies. Later, the settlers began to consume it, acquiring it from the Indians. Tobacco cultivation quickly spread to Brazil, especially to the north-east, and to other European countries such as France and Portugal. In just one century, tobacco became known all over the world, having been used initially for medicinal purposes and later to make cigars and cigarettes (SEFRINI, 1995).

Currently, the production and commercialisation of tobacco and its derivatives is carried out in more than fifty countries. The largest producers are China, Brazil, India, Zimbabwe and Indonesia, which account for around 70 per cent of world tobacco production (DEPARTAMENTO DE ESTUDOS SOCIOECONÔMICO RURAIS, 2003).

Since 2007, Brazil has ranked second in tobacco production, accounting for 26.9 per cent of world exports. In comparative figures, production in 2007 was 59% higher than in 2000. It currently exports around 85% of its annual production (DEPARTAMENTO DE ESTUDOS SOCIOECONÔMICO RURAIS, 2009). The production of good quality leaf requires extensive use of agrochemicals and large-scale use has caused damage to the health of farmers and their families, as well as to the ecosystem, contributing to the loss of biodiversity (SCHOENHALS, 2009).

In the Northeast, production is independent, with few agreements with companies. In Alagoas, almost 132,000 people have tobacco as their main income and Arapiraca is the main producer of rope and leaf tobacco, the latter being exported (NADIR, 2007).

In the north-east, tobacco is sown in mid-May, transplanted in June and harvested between August and September. Once the seedlings have been sown, the pest and disease control phase becomes intensive. Various types of pesticides are used during the tobacco leaf production cycle. After the harvest period, the leaves are tied up and stretched out on clotheslines to dry, and only then is the stalk of the tobacco leaf removed so that it can later be rolled up and put up for sale or stored (DEPARTAMENTO DE ESTUDOS SOCIOECONÔMICO RURAIS, 2003a). Throughout production, tobacco growers in Arapiraca are exposed to pesticides due to the lack of personal protective equipment (PPE) (NASCIMENTO, 2011).

Brazilian tobacco growing has occupied a prominent place on the world market due to its large production of tobacco leaves from this *commodity* (DEPARTAMENTO DE ESTUDOS SOCIOECONÔMICO RURAIS, 2003a; 2009). This is a worrying factor if we consider the emergence of health problems related to handling tobacco leaves and the intensive use of agrochemicals in this crop. Working conditions and the negative influence on the mental health of tobacco farmers and their families are also factors that contribute to the emergence of health problems in this population (CAMPAIGNING FOR TOBACCO FREE KIDS, 2001).

3.2 Pesticides: a brief historical review

Primitive civilisations, essentially rural, were dedicated to agriculture and livestock farming using simple technologies, at a time when there was no distinction between producer and consumer (HERRERA, 1990). Practices aimed at satisfying basic needs were organised to keep food compatible with the demands of this society.

From this perspective, the history of ancient Rome records the use of smoke from burning sulphur to control aphids, as well as salt to prevent weeds. Arsenic mixed with water was used by the Chinese to control insects at the beginning of the 19th century (BOHMONT, 1981), which was also a time when there was a need to reduce crop pests. It is recorded that until 1930 the substances used for this type of control were of organic origin (BULL; HATHAWAY, 1986). From World War II onwards, most of these substances became synthetic, and during this period Dichloro-Diphenyl-Trichloroethane (DDT) and organophosphorus compounds were used as chemical weapons, to which longer carbon chains and combinations of elements such as phosphorus, sulphur, nitrogen and chlorine were added (BULL; HATHAWAY, 1986).

With the end of the war, world agriculture underwent profound transformations, beginning with the "Green Revolution", which led to profound changes in traditional agriculture. The globalisation of the economy, the emergence of large companies and the industrial revolution that took place during that period supported the increase in agricultural products, resulting in a reduction in rural labour and the maximisation of monoculture cultivation (CHAIM, 1999). Agricultural production based on technological innovations and investments in irrigation techniques, combined with the intensive use of mechanisation and industrial inputs, resulted in the intensive use of pesticides and fertilisers. This practice has had a negative impact on the environment and human health (OLIVEIRA-SILVA et al.; GARCIA, 2001; SPADOTTO et al., 2004). These changes associated with ageing populations have led to new patterns of morbidity and mortality, including a significant increase in the occurrence of diseases such as cardiovascular and mental illness in rural workers (POSSAS & TRAPÉ, 1983).

Chemical products used to control pests have been given various names such as pesticides, pesticides and pesticides. However, in Brazil, since the promulgation of the 1988 Constitution, this group of products has been called pesticides (Federal Law No. 7.802 of 11 July 1989, regulated by Decree No. 4.074 of January 2002) (PERES, 2003). After the "Green Revolution", technological models were introduced in Brazil, and on this occasion the "National Agricultural Development Plan" was created, which linked the release of "rural credit" to the compulsory purchase of pesticides, a context that led to the growth of the synthetic pesticide industry and the dependence of agriculture on these compounds (FERREIRA, 1999). Since then, this activity has been geared towards commercial production in order to meet the needs of an ever-growing population, which, according to the United Nations, will be approximately 7.9 billion people by 2025 (INTERNATIONAL LABOUR ORGANISATION, 2001).

3.3 Classification of pesticides

Pesticides are used in various types of activity and correspond to a wide variety of chemical substances, some of which are of biological origin and others synthetic. From this perspective, they can be classified according to various aspects, ranging from the type of pest they control and the chemical structure of the active ingredients, to the effects they can have on health and the environment. In terms of purpose of use, they are divided into acaricides, avicides, bactericides, fungicides, herbicides, insecticides, among others (MELNIKOV, 1971).

Considering the chemical group, they are classified as insecticides, fungicides and herbicides. Insecticides are subdivided into chlorinated hydrocarbons (e.g. Aldrim, chlorodane), organophosphates (Diazinon, parathion, malathion), carbamates (Carbaryl, methomyl), pyrethroids (Pyrethrin), neonicotinoids (Imidacloprid). Fungicides in Thiocarbamates (Ferbam), Mercurials (Ceresan), Strobilurin (Azoxystrobin) and Herbicides in Phenoxyalkyl acids (2,4-D,); Triazines (Atrazine,); Phenylureas (fluometuron); Aliphatic acids (Dalapon); Carbamates (Butylate); Dinitroanilines (Trifularim); Dipyridyls (Paraquat); Amides (Propanil); Benzoics (Amiben) (BRADY, 1989) and glycine derivatives (Glyphosate). According to the World Health Organisation, the recommended and generally used classification is the toxicological one, which can be defined as: "classification of technical products and formulations taking into account their toxicological aspects" (BRASIL, 1998), expressed in Average Lethal Dose (ALD50) values, orally. The product's active ingredient is measured in terms of kilograms of live weight, i.e. what is needed to kill 50% of the population of rats or other test animals.

Thus, container labels must contain a coloured band indicating their toxicological class (SIQUEIRA; KRUSE, 2008). Accordingly, pesticides are grouped into classes as described in Table 1.

Table 1 - Toxicological classification of pesticides according to DL50

Toxicological class	Groups	DL 50	Dose capable of killing an adult person	Colour
Ia	Extremely toxic	< 5 mg/kg	1 pinch = a	Red

			few drops	
Ib	Highly toxic	5- 50 mg/kg	A few drops = 1 teaspoon	Yellow
II	Medium toxic	50- 500 mg/kg	1 teaspoon = 2 tablespoons	Blue
III	Low toxicity	500-5000 mg/kg	2 tablespoons =1 cup	Green
-	Very low toxicity	5000 mg/kg or +	1 glass = 1 litre	-

Source: Adapted from OPS, 1996. WHO, 2009.

The lethal dose classification is a criterion that only measures the acute toxicity of a chemical substance on animal species and does not indicate possible physiological, biochemical and histological alterations in these organisms resulting from prolonged exposure, whether through the absorption of small doses, continued or not, known as chronic toxicity.

It can also be classified according to its formulation, which can be solid (dry powder, wettable powder, granules) or liquid (water-soluble, emulsifiable). This condition is important when considering the route of absorption and the environmental conditions in which the product is being handled (SILVA & FAY, 2004). There are currently more than three hundred active ingredients, which, when combined with other substances, result in more than two thousand formulations available on the Brazilian market. These principles can also be associated according to their action and chemical group (PAN-AMERICAN HEALTH ORGANISATION/WORLD HEALTH ORGANISATION, 1996). Among the best-selling pesticides are herbicides (Toxicological Classes II and III), insecticides (Classes I and II) and fungicides (Class III) (SINDICATO NACIONAL DA INDÚSTRIA DE PRODUTOS PARA DEFESA AGRÍCOLA, 2001; DEWAR, 2007).

3.4 Human health and pesticides

Pesticides are chemical substances or mixtures used to prevent, destroy or repel pathogens or animal or plant life (Federal Law No. 7.802 of 11 July 1989). They were introduced to the market with the aim of increasing the availability of food for the world's population, improving the yield, quality and aesthetics of the products produced (OERKE & DEHNE, 2004; COOPER & DOBSON, 2007). Released in large quantities into the environment, these products ended up reaching non-target organisms, which contributed to the emergence of some negative side effects on human health and the environment (HAMILTON, 2004).

The Brazilian market now consumes 84% of the pesticides sold in Latin America. Growth has been so significant that between 1990 and 2008 this market grew by 140%, generating figures of around 6 billion dollars (PELAEZ, 2011). There are currently more than 65,000 chemical products classified as pesticides (MECDAD et al., 2011).

Linked to the disorganised growth of this market and the lack of preparation of the workers who handle these substances have been the growing consequences expressed by SINITOX (National Toxic-Pharmacological Information System - Ministry of Health/FIOCRUZ), which recorded around 62,000 poisonings from agricultural pesticides between 1999 and 2009 (BRASIL, 2011). It is estimated that for every reported case there are 50 unreported cases (PERES et. al.; RECENA, 2005). This fact is part of the magnitude of the public health problem that exists in the country and which led to the mandatory reporting of these events in all Brazilian states from January 2011 (BOMBARD, 2011).

According to Bochner (2007), in Brazil, poisoning is recorded by two systems: SINITOX (linked to FIOCRUZ and whose purpose is to provide clinical guidance to health professionals) and SINAN (Sistema de Informação de Agravos de Notificação - Notifiable Diseases Information System), linked directly to the Ministry of Health, with the aim of notifying this problem (pesticide poisoning) and others. However, these databases only provide information on cases of acute poisoning, which have immediate effects, and do not have official records on the chronic effects caused by these substances.

In the Northeast, the number of poisoning cases reported in SINITOX and the incidence of deaths from pesticide poisoning is high, possibly because it is associated with the large number of suicide attempts in relation to the total number of poisonings (BOMBARD, 2011).

Poisoning can be acute, sub-chronic or chronic. The latter is characterised by a delayed onset over months or years with small or moderate exposure to toxic products or multiple products, triggering irreversible damage (STOPELLI & MAGALHÃES, 2005).

According to Nascimento (2011), pyrethroids, neonicotinoids and organophosphates (OFs) are among the chemical groups most commonly used in tobacco growing in the municipality of Arapiraca, with methamidophos and chlorpyrifos standing out because they are banned in Brazil (ANVISA). These substances were used in high concentrations in World War II as war weaponry due to their high toxicity, and were known at the time as "mustard gas" and "nerve gas" (PAN-AMERICAN HEALTH ORGANISATION, 1996).

OFs are powerful inhibitors of cholinesterases, key enzymes for the central and peripheral nervous system (COSTA et al., 2005). These cause a higher prevalence of poisoning symptoms in farmers who apply them than in those who don't (SMIT, 2003). In the literature there are records indicating that several OFs are mutagenic (MATSUSHITA; MATSUI; MATSUSHITA et al., 2005).

Pyrethroids were introduced into the environment in the 19th century, derived from *chrysanthemums* (MILLER, 2002). This insecticide acts on the sodium channels in the membrane of neurons, allowing them to remain open longer than necessary (MACAN, 2006). The toxic signs triggered by the neuroexcitatory effects commonly produce the "T" intoxication syndrome (as it produces tremor), nervous disorders, salivation, convulsions and potent sympathetic activation. Dermal contamination can cause irritation, including flushing and oedema of the skin and paresthesia (SODERLUND et al., 2001; MACAN, 2006).

OF compounds can be absorbed via the skin, respiratory and digestive routes, especially when personal protective equipment (PPE) is not used (ANDRADE, 2001). After absorption, this chemical group and the product of its biotransformation are rapidly distributed throughout the body and the most lipophilic compounds reach important concentrations in nervous tissue (CALDAS et al., 2000). This substance irreversibly inhibits cholinesterases and promotes the accumulation of the neurotransmitter acetylcholine in the synaptic clefts, overstimulating muscarinic and nicotinic receptors and triggering parasympathomimetic effects (PAN-AMERICAN HEALTH ORGANISATION/WORLD HEALTH ORGANISATION, 1996), i.e. in the autonomic and central nervous system, exocrine glands and neuromuscular motor plate.

The symptoms caused by OFs when the disease turns into intoxication can be drowsiness, headaches, loss of concentration, fatigue, mental confusion, emotional lability, hypertension, dyspnoea, sweating and diarrhoea. The behavioural effects resulting from the use of these compounds are worrying given the variety of psychiatric sequelae such as depression and schizophrenia (COSTA, 2005). These mental illnesses can lead farmers and their families to commit suicide. Post-intoxication depression can be observed in suicidal and non-suicidal people exposed to pesticides (CALDAS et al., 2000). As an example of environmental exposure, after a disaster in Mississippi in the USA, OF was found in the drinking water of more than half the population (REHNER, 2000), a fact that may be associated with the symptoms of depression that these people showed.

The symptoms of intoxication can be initial, such as sweating, salivation, tearing, dizziness, blurred vision and late effects such as vomiting, muscle tremors and difficulty breathing. Late action occurs through neurotoxicity with late-onset peripheral neuropathy, paresthesias and motor paralyses in the lower limbs.

A study by Salvi et al. (2003) identified neuropsychiatric and extrapyramidal symptoms in individuals chronically exposed to organophosphates. The population studied showed normal levels of acetylcholinesterase, highlighting the need for other parameters to biomonitor the consequences of this type of exposure.

According to Ray and Richards (2001) very low doses of organophosphates, when they trigger cholinergic signals, produce various effects in experimental animals such as low learning capacity, alterations in the ear labyrinth and even slowing down nerve conduction. They also claim that other more sensitive brain proteins are the target of these actions, not just acetylcholinesterase. Indicating that the mechanism of action of these compounds is not necessarily via inhibition of acetylcholinesterase.

According to He et al. (2002) exposure to an organophosphate, either alone or in combination with pyrethroids for two hours, will produce an acetylcholinesterase inhibition effect similar to organophosphates when not combined because they are more potent than pyrethroids.

The physiological lesions resulting from acute intoxication begin to appear after a fortnight because the disease produces alterations in liver enzymes, kidney damage and even cardiac arrhythmias identified through complementary tests. These consequences are probably due to the elimination process of OFs, which occurs through hepatic metabolism and oxidative metabolites, most of which are excreted via the kidneys. Difficult to characterise, the clinical picture can become apparent after years of exposure (SOARES et al., 2003).

In the literature, there are also records indicating that several OFs are mutagenic (MATSUSHITA; MATSUI; MATSUSHITA et al., 2005). They also have an immunosuppressive effect on humans and animals (NEWCOMBE, 1992a).

Table 2 - Effects of exposure to organophosphate pesticides

EFFECTOR MECHANISMS	SYSTEMS AND ORGANS	SIGNS AND SYMPTOMS
	Respiratory system	Bronchoconstriction, cough - Bronchial hypersecretion - Oedema pulmonary, cyanosis
	Cardiovascular system	-Bradicardia , hypotension
MUSCARINICS		- QT prolongation
	Urinary system	- Polaciuria -Incontinence urinary

	Digestive system	-Colic abs -Nausea , vomiting, anorexia -Diarrhoea , tenesmus -Incontinence faecal
	Eyes	- Myosis - Decreased visual acuity
	Glands	- Increased sweating - Increased tearing - Increased salivation
NICOTINIC	**Striated muscle**	- Fasciculations -Cramps , hypotonia
	Sympathetic ganglia	-Pallor , tachycardia -Hypertension arterial
		- Hyperthermia, tachycardia
SYSTEM NERVOUS CENTRE		- Lability emotional - Depression, ataxia - Apathy, headache - Anxiety, asthenia

		- Coma with abolished reflexes - EEG changes - Cheyne-Stokes respiration - Convulsions, confusion - Excitement, depression of the respiratory and circulatory centres
MANIFESTATIONS NON-CHOLINERGIC		- Arrhythmias cardiac -Neuropathy peripheral -Toxicity pulmonary

Source: JUNIOR et al (1999).

Neonicotinoids are a new class of insecticides that have been used extensively, accounting for around a fifth of the global insecticide market (TOMIZAWA, 2005). Similar in structure and action to nicotine, they are agonists of the nicotinic acetylcholine receptor (nAChR) and are much more toxic to insects than to mammals, due to the differences in their interactions (TOMIZAWA, 2005). However, it still has toxicological effects on humans. These are the same as those of nicotine, such as nausea, fatigue, muscle weakness, headaches and others (ENRIQUEZ, 2003).

The literature consistently describes the immediate intoxication process of many agrochemicals, but still leaves gaps regarding chronic lesions. From this perspective, some pathologies that develop over the long term stand out, such as skin diseases, teratogenesis, effects on human reproduction (CLAPP et al., 2008; BILA, 2007) and cancers such as lung cancer, breast cancer, testicular cancer, thyroid cancer, prostate cancer, ovarian cancer and cancers of the haematopoietic system (non-Hodgkin's lymphoma, leukaemia and multiple myeloma) (PIMENTEL, 1996).

According to Londres et al. (2011), cancer cases in children have tripled and births of babies with malformations have quadrupled in Argentina in the last decade. (2008), being a farmer increases the risk of developing cancer when compared to the general population. Studies report that in chronic intoxication, neurobehavioural disorders are recorded from general symptoms such as insomnia, sleepwalking, excessive sleep, anxiety, delayed reactions, difficulty concentrating and a variety of neuropsychiatric sequelae, emotional lability, language disorders, apathy, irritability, hallucinations, delusions, tremors, schizophrenic reactions, EEG alterations, peripheral neuropathy, paresthesia, hyporeflexia, impaired neuro-motor coordination and depression (ECOBICHON, 2001).

The widespread use of pesticides by rural workers has resulted in a wide range of health problems, as well as increasing the risk of mental health problems when compared to the urban population (FARIA et al., 2000). The association of mental illness with crops and pesticides has also been reported in the literature, such as the case of Venâncio Aires (RS), which associated the handling of tobacco leaves and the use of organophosphates with the prevalence of suicide, where a rate of almost 37 suicides per 100,000 inhabitants was found (FALK, 1996). The literature also deals with the relationship between the prevalence of poisoning, suicide attempts and exposure to organophosphate and carbamate pesticides (SOARES; ALMEIDA; SAVI et al., 2003).

The intensive and multi-chemical use of pesticides has worried the scientific community. Related to these factors is the lack of skilled labour to handle these products and the lack of adequate supervision of their marketing (PESSOA, 2002). The interactions of various chemical compounds, impurities and "inert" substances simultaneously during work (SILVA, 2000; SOARES et al., 2003) are still underestimated factors, a fact that has resulted in fragilities ranging from health problems to environmental imbalances, harming not only humans, but also fauna and flora.

Regarding the conditions of contact with pesticides, there may be modified interactions due to high temperatures, greater contact due to not observing the wind when applying pesticides to the crop. With regard to labour effort, there is an increase in physical effort with a consequent increase in pulmonary ventilation and blood circulation. In addition to these aspects, agricultural activities include the preparation and application of pesticides, further exposing rural workers and potentially causing acute, subacute or chronic intoxication (SILVA, 2005). The process of acute exposure to a chemical product occurs in large doses over a short period of time and varies in terms of intensity (mild to severe) (Chart 2).

Chronic exposure is related to prolonged contact of months to years and low concentrations. The clinical characterisation of these episodes is more difficult, as they usually come from multiple contaminants, a common case in agriculture, where cause and effect are not recognised. Data from the literature shows a number of alterations resulting from chronic intoxication, including immunological, genetic, haematopoietic, hepatic, respiratory, endocrine, cardiovascular, genitourinary, reproductive, gastrointestinal, skin, eye, allergy reactions, malformations and behavioural alterations (COLOSSO et al., 2003; ALAVANJA et al., 2004) (Table 3 and Table 4).

Table 3 - Effects of exposure to pesticides from the main pesticide groups according to action and chemical groups to which they belong

Classification (Action)	**Chemical group**	**Trade name**	**Acute poisoning**	**Chronic intoxication**
INSECTICIDES	Organophosphates and carbamates	Malation Paration Fenitrotion Benomil Carbendazima	Weakness Abdominal colic Vomit Muscle spasms Seizure	Delayed neurological effects Chromosomal changes Contact dermatitis
	Organochlorines	Aldrin	Nausea Vomit	Cardiac arrhythmias Kidney damage

		DDT	Involuntary muscle contractions	Peripheral neuropathies
	Synthetic pyrethroids	Deltametrina, Permethrin	Irritation of the conjunctivae Sneezing Excitement Convulsion	Allergies Bronchial asthma Irritation mucous membranes Hypersensitivity
FUNGICIDES	Dithiocarbamates	Mancozeb Metiram	Dizziness Vomit Muscle tremors Dor de head	Respiratory allergies Dermatitis Disease Parkinson Cancers
	Fentalamides	Captafol Captan		Teratogenesis
	Dinitrophenols and Pentachlorophenol	Bromophenexim DNOC	Difficulty breathing Hyperthermia Convulsion	Cancers Chloroacnes
HERBICIDES	Phenoxyacetic s	CMPP 2,4-D	Loss of appetite Motion sickness Vomit Muscle fasciculation	Induction of liver enzyme production Cancers Teratogenesis
	Dipyridyl	Paraquat Diquat	Nosebleed Weakness Fainting Conjunctivitis	Liver damage Contact dermatitis Pulmonary fibrosis

Source: WHO, 1990; OPS/WHO, 1996.

Another important aspect of pesticide poisoning involves exposure to multiple compounds. Interactions between pesticides occur between themselves and organic biological systems where unknown toxic behaviours can lead to various health effects for the exposed worker. So far, what is available is only data on some synergistic responses resulting from the interactions of these chemicals used in the daily lives of rural workers (WHO, 1981).

It should be emphasised that the combination of product mixtures occurs both in the field and in the companies where these substances are produced, either directly or indirectly. According to Sindag (2003), mixtures of active ingredients such as 2,4-D + Diazinon (herbicide), Benalaxy + Mancozeb (fungicide) or Deltamethrin + Triazophos (insecticide) was freely commercialised without the necessary studies. Exposure to mixtures of chemical substances can have independent, synergistic or antagonistic effects, which affect the potential deleterious effects of each on human health. It is known that the human body's responses to pesticide-related activities can be influenced by characteristics such as smoking, alcoholism and nutritional status, which makes the assessment of chemical mixtures even more complex (SILVA, 2005).

Describing the toxicity of multiple exposures to pesticides and various chemical products is a major challenge for the scientific community. This situation not only affects farmers, but also workers in the manufacturing and service industries, mining, laboratories and others. Little research has documented the effects of this type of exposure (Table 4).

Table 4 - Effects of chronic exposure to multiple pesticides

BODY/ SYSTEM	EFFECT
NERVOUS SYSTEM	Astheno-vegetative syndrome Vegetative polyneuritis Radiculitis Encephalopathies - Dysencephalitis Vegetative vascular dystonia Cerebral sclerosis Retrobulbar neuritis with visual acuity Retinal angiopathy
RESPIRATORY SYSTEM	Chronic tracheitis - Pneumofibrosis initial - Pulmonary emphysema - Bronchial asthma
	Chronic toxic myocarditis Chronic coronary insufficiency Hypertension - Hypotension
CARDIOVASCULAR	

SYSTEM	
LIVER	Chronic hepatitis - Cholecystitis Impairment of detoxification and other functions
RINS	Albuminuria - Nicturia - Urea, Nitrogen and Creatinine, Clearance
TREATMENT GASTROINTESTINAL	Chronic gastritis - Duodenitis - Ulcers -Chronic colitis (haemorrhagic, spastic and polypoid formations) Hypersecretion and Hyperacidity Motor impairment
SYSTEM H IN ETHICAL ATOPOI	Leucopenia - Reticulocytes Lymphocytes - Eosinopenia - Monocytosis - Changes In haemoglobin
SKIN	Dermatitis - Eczema
EYES	Conjunctivitis - Blepharitis

Source: Kaloyanova & Simeonova (1977).

It has been recognised for some time that there are adverse effects resulting from this type of exposure (KALOYANOVA, 1983), although without defining a specific group of pesticides, but rather the synergistic action of pesticides. Table 4 shows the diversity of effects on the different systems of the human organism resulting from chronic exposure to the combined use of multiple pesticides. This situation constitutes a public health problem.

The use of the most diverse formulations has become routine in agriculture. As these become available on the agrochemical market, more unanswered questions arise about the health-disease process, making it necessary to seek solutions. Occupational monitoring through laboratory tests is one of the few tools available to screen for pre-complication alterations and is of paramount importance for the promotion, prevention and diagnosis of diseases caused by agrochemicals.

3.5 Pesticide use and human biological monitoring

Biological monitoring has been an important ally in pesticide research. Carried out using biomarkers, biomonitoring from a practical point of view has been used in risk assessment (risk identification) for the health of an exposed group, dose-response analysis, exposure assessment (risk quantification), risk characterisation, as well as in the diagnosis of diseases related to an individual's exposure (AITIO, 1999). In short, they result in information that can support the modification of any practices or situations that occur at work, favouring the prevention of health problems.

According to Groopman and Kensler (1999), human biomonitoring involves the identification of biomarkers in body fluids, cells and tissues with the aim of assessing exposure and effects, predicting the risk of disease and providing objective measures to determine the effectiveness of interventions in order to reduce exposure and risk. It is also defined in the field of human health as indicators of normal biological processes, pathogenic processes or pharmacological responses to a therapeutic intervention (BIOMARKERS DEFINITIONS WORKING GROUP, 2001).

In the mid-1970s, biomarkers became available almost exponentially, from around 150 tests in the three-year period 19771979 to more than 5,200 in the 1990s (PIVETTA, 2001).

At the beginning of the 1990s, biomarkers marked the period as one of the most promising approaches to signalling specific exposures or stages of the disease, but despite the advances, their quantity is still insufficient for the existing demands (BONASSI et al., 2001). One of the main functions of biomarkers is to provide an early warning of significant biological effects (LAM & GRAY, 2001). In this process, knowing the sequences of events triggered and breaking down these pathways is one of the great challenges for modern epidemiology and toxicology.

According to Famer et al. (2003) and Scherer (2005), biomarkers are commonly classified as exposure (divided into internal and external dose), effect (generally early biological effects, signalling potential damage) and susceptibility (individual factors that alter the risk of disease). They are especially useful in assessing progressive diseases where symptoms appear long after exposure (WARD, 1999). Some of them are highly specific, i.e. they respond only to a chemical substance or a group, such as the enzyme aminolevulinic acid dehydrogenase (inhibited by lead), and can be extremely sensitive (SELANDER, 1970).

For Larsen (1995), the chain of events in exposure includes the external and internal dose ("absorbed dose"), biologically understood as the effective dose (target dose), which leads to the onset of the biological health effect. This must be understood as a multifactorial process, i.e. taking into account age, gender, ethnicity, environmental exposure, physiological and nutritional conditions and hormonal status, which can modify the entire response context (VAINIO, 1999).

According to Shugart (2000), examples of biomarkers include glycosylated haemoglobin, lymphocyte count, sperm count, macrophage activity, red blood cell count, cotinine (nicotine), acetylcholinesterase activity (organophosphates), retinol (b-carotene), gamma-glutamyl transferase (liver toxins) and creatine kinase (muscle trauma).

Biomarkers of effect reflect physiological and morphological changes in cells and tissues, without necessarily changing their function, and may involve responses from biochemical measurements (WARD, 1999).

In addition to these measurements, normal haematological parameters are fundamental when it comes to assessing a population's state of health and standard of living. Since the 1970s, blood components have been recognised as promising biomarkers for insecticide toxicity (BELL et al., 1972).

Biomonitoring depends not only on the biomarkers, but also on the reference values of the kits used for analysis, since exposed individuals must be compared using the same parameter with the population under study or by environmental situation to the xenobiotics assessed (AITIO, 1994). These values have to be determined for each country and/or region, taking into account factors that may affect the assessment, such as diet, location, housing, habits specific to the region, environmental pollution and others (BERTAZZI et al., 1988).

In order to make it possible to interpret the results of biomarker analyses, Brazil's regulatory standard included the maximum permitted values (Maximum Permitted Biological Index - IBMP), which it is assumed that the majority of workers will not show harmful effects when they are below these values. Reference values for these parameters have also been established (MINISTÉRIO DO TRABALHO, 1994), while there are adequate parameters for each region that is monitored.

In public health, biomonitoring is an inseparable part of occupational and environmental health surveillance due to its multiple and ecological nature (MACHADO, 1997), which interdisciplinarily connects the biological with the environmental, linking the individual with the collective, defining and redefining risk groups in the health-disease process (PIVETTA, 1999).

Based on the premise that physiological parameters are fundamental for assessing the state of health of individuals and the population and that they can be bio-markers of exposure to pesticides, the aim of this study was to characterise the blood count and serum biochemical profile of tobacco farmers exposed to pesticides in the rural area of Arapiraca (AL).

CHAPTER 4

MATERIAL AND METHODS

4.1 Definition and characterisation of the study area

The study area was the rural area of Arapiraca, a municipality in the central region of Alagoas and the second most populous city in the state. The estimated population for 2009 was approximately 210,000 inhabitants, with 19% living in rural areas (Chart 5).

Table 5 - General information about Arapiraca

Area, population and tobacco production	
Area	351 kilometres^2
Estimated population	210,521 inhabitants
Urban population	170.522 (81%)
Rural population	39.999 (19%)
Annual tobacco production	4081 tonnes
Area planted with tobacco	3580 hectares

Source: Brazilian Foundation of Geography and Statistics - IBGE, 2009.

4.2 Type of Study

This was an analytical cross-sectional study. The analysis and description of variables relating to the characteristics of the population and occupational exposure to pesticides involved data collection using a semi-structured questionnaire.

4.3 Sampling

This study selected 200 subjects for convenience and 166 of them took part in the study. They were given a haemogram and serum biochemical tests, as well as answering a semi-structured questionnaire.

4.3.1 Ethical issues

The study was approved by the Oswaldo Cruz Foundation's Research Ethics Committee under opinion no. 205/09. The participants in this study were informed before the interview about the study's objectives and those who agreed to take part signed the Free and Informed Consent Form, in accordance with Resolution 196/96 of the National Health Council/Ministry of Health (ANNEX A), which restricted the use of biological material for research into the effects of exposure to pesticides.

4.4 Sampling criteria

4.4.1 Inclusion criteria

Tobacco workers who had also applied pesticides for at least 12 months and who lived in the locality being researched took part in the study.

4.4.2 Exclusion criteria

Tobacco farmers who did not sign the Informed Consent Form, as well as those under 18 years of age and workers who had not applied pesticides for at least 12 months were excluded from taking part in the study. The tests of some of the participants were excluded because the laboratory where the analyses were carried out would not release the results because they were too high.

4.5 Data collection through a questionnaire

Data was collected in two stages. The first took place during the period when the tobacco farmers were applying pesticides, when the exposure assessment questionnaire was used. The questionnaire contains closed and open questions to assess occupational and environmental exposure to pesticides. The interview lasted approximately 25 minutes.

This instrument was applied in the selected properties before the peripheral venipunctures. The variables contained in the questionnaire were the following: socioeconomic, demographic, characteristics of the work process, characteristics of exposure to pesticides and nicotine, prevention and health conditions.

Blood samples were collected a few days after the questionnaires were administered. The blood samples were handled in accordance with ethical standards and meeting ethical and biosafety criteria. Data collection took place between August and September 2011.

4.6 Blood collection

Blood was collected only after signing the Free and Informed Consent Form and being interviewed with a questionnaire. The procedure was carried out by venepuncture in the "fall" period (a few days after the pesticide application), using a syringe or vacunteiner, in three tubes containing EDTA and a dry tube.

4.6.1 Tests

4.6.1.1 Serum biochemistry

Serum biochemistry tests were carried out at the Arapiraca Municipal Health Laboratory, immediately after blood collection. The analyses were carried out on the Abbott Aeroset c 8000 automated device (Abbott Company, USA) using kits from the French company ELITECh, according to the manufacturer's recommendations. The parameters analysed were glucose, urea, creatinine, uric acid, total proteins and fractions (albumins, globulins, A/G ratio), albumin, cholesterol, triglycerides, phosphorus, HDL cholesterol, LDL cholesterol, bilirubin, oxalacetic transaminase (TGO), pyruvic transaminase

(TGP), alkaline phosphatase, gamma glutamyl transferase (GGT), amylase, lactate dehydrogenase (LDH), serum calcium, serum iron, potassium, sodium, magnesium, lipase and ferritin. Table 6 shows the reference values for each variable investigated.

Table 6 - Reference values for serum biochemical parameters analysed in rural workers from Arapiraca (AL)

EXAMINATION	UNIT	MAN	WOMAN
1 Glucose	mg/dL	60-110	
2 Urea	mg/dL	13-43	
3 Creatinine	mg/dL	0,6-1,2	
4 Uric acid	mg/dL	3,5-7,2	2,6-6,00
5 Alkaline phosphatase	U/L	40-150	
6 GGT	U/L	1,0-38	
7 Amylase	U/L	1,0-90	
8 LDH	U/L	235 - 470	
9 Calcium	mg/dl	8,6-10,3	
10 Serum iron	Ug/dL	50-175	
11 Potassium	Eq/L	3,8-5,6	
12 Lipase	U.I/L	1-59	
13 Ferritin	ng/mL	24 - 336	11-307
14 Sodium	Eq/L	138-145	
15AST (TGO)	UK/mL	4-40	
16 ALT (TGP)	UK/mL	4-36	
17 Cholesterol	mg/dL	Desirable < 200 Borderline up to 260	

		High> 260
18 Triglycerides	mg/dL	Up to 200
19 HDL - cholesterol	mg/dL	Desirable >60 Acceptable 41 - 59 Low=40
20 LDL - cholesterol	mg/dL	Desirable >130 Borderline 131 - 159 High> 160
21Proteins totals	g/dL	6-8
22 Albumin	g/dL	3,6-4,9
23 Globulin	g/dL	1,9-3,1
24 A/G ratio	g/dL	1,4-2,3
25 Total bilirubin	mg/dL	0,2- 1,2
26 Bilirubin direct	mg/dL	0,1-0,5
27 Bilirubin indirect	mg/dL	0,28-1,2
28 Phosphorus	Eq/L	2,7 - 4,5

Source: Abbott Aero set (USA).

4.6.1.2 Blood count

The blood count was carried out at the Arapiraca Municipal Health Laboratory, using the Cell - Dyn 3700 automated device (Abbott Company, USA) using the electrical impedance method and flow cytometry. Red cell parameters were assessed (haematocrit, haemoglobin - HGB, RBC, mean corpuscular volume - MCV, mean corpuscular haemoglobin - MCH, mean corpuscular haemoglobin concentration - MCHC), leucogram (leucocytes, rods, segmented, lymphocytes, monocytes, eosinophils, basophils, myelocytes, metamyelocytes), haematoscopy and platelet count. Table 7 shows the reference values for men and women.

Table 7 - Blood count reference values for rural workers in Arapiraca (AL)

ERYTHROGRAMME	**REFERENCE VALUES MAN (%)**	**REFERENCE VALUES WOMAN(%)**
1 Haematocrit	40-54	36-47
2 Haemoglobin - HGB	13,5-18	11,5-16
3 Haematia	4,5-6,5	
4 Mean corpuscular volume - MCV	80-100	
5Hemoglobin mean corpuscular	27-32	

blood count - MCH		
6Concentration haemoglobin- CHCM	32-36	
7 Platelet count	140 - 400 (mil/mm $)^3$	140 - 400 (mil/mm $)^3$

LEUCOGRAM	**REFERENCE VALUES (MM $)^3$**
1 Leucocytes	5000- 10000
2 sticks	150-500
3 Segmented	2700 - 6200
4 Lymphocytes	1000-3500
5 Monocytes	150-800
6 Eosinophils	100-600
7 Basophils	0-100
8 Myelocytes	0
9 Metamyelocytes	0 - 100

Source: Abboatt (USA).

4. 7Data analysis

The data obtained in the survey was stored in Microsoft Excel spreadsheets, version 2010. The demographic, socioeconomic, working conditions and worker exposure variables were analysed using SPSS version 20.0. Categorical variables were analysed using the Chi-squared test and continuous variables using Student's t-test and ANOVA. The significance level used was 95% (p-value <0.05).

The analyses were approached in such a way as to allow individuals to be grouped by exposure, socioeconomic and demographic characteristics. First, the data was analysed taking into account socioeconomic, demographic and exposure variables such as location, gender, age, ethnicity, schooling, working hours, tobacco consumption, alcohol consumption, type of contact with pesticides, reported symptoms and type of pesticide. The individuals were then grouped according to gender using Student's t-test to compare means and Pearson's chi-squared test for frequencies. All the biochemical and haematological analyses were approached by gender, comparing the means using Student's t-test.

CHAPTER 1

CHAPTER 5

RESULTS

5.1 Socio-economic, demographic and occupational profiles of tobacco workers

Initially, a descriptive study was carried out to identify the sociodemographic characteristics of the population. Interviews and blood samples were taken from 166 rural tobacco workers who apply pesticides living in Arapiraca - AL. Some important demographic characteristics of the group studied are shown in Table 1.

The rural workers in this study were mainly pesticide applicators. Their average age was 43.24 (±12.42), with 67 (40.4%) women and 99 (59.6%) men. There was no significant difference in age in relation to the gender of the rural worker. As for ethnicity, 93 (56%) declared themselves to be mixed race, 23 (13.9%) white, 47 (28.3%) black and 01 (0.6%) Indian, with 02 (1.2%) not answering, which showed that the highest frequency was mixed race and black (Table 1).

Table 1 - Demographic data of the study population

Sex		**F (%)**
Men		99(59,6)
Women		67(40,4)
Age		
Average	43,24	
Standard deviation (SD)	12,426	
Ethnicity		**F(%)**
White		23(14,0)
Mestizo		93(56,7)
Black		47(28,7)
Indian		1(0,6)
Total		164(100)

Source: Author of this dissertation, 2012.

Table 2 shows the frequency of farmers in relation to the study locations and ethnicity. The Pau D'arco locality had a higher frequency of blacks (54.5%) than the other localities, while Capim and Mundo Novo (69.4%), Canaã (57.1%) and Batingas (74.2%) had a higher frequency of mixed-race farmers.

Table 2 - Frequency of farmers in relation to ethnicity and location of study

Location	**Ethnicity**		
	White	**Black**	**Mestizo**
	F (%)	**F(%)**	**F(%)**
	6 (12,2%)	9(18,4%)	3(69,4%)

Capim and Mundo Novo			4
Canaan	6 (21,4%)	6(21,4%)	16(57,1%)
Pau D'arco	5 (9,1%)	30(54,5%)	20(36,4%)
Batingas	6 (19,4%)	2(6,5%)	23(74,2%)

Source: Author of this dissertation, 2012.

As shown in figure 2, most of the group who took part in the survey had little schooling, since regardless of gender, 103 (62.1%) had not completed primary school, 38 (22.9) had not completed secondary school, 12 (7.2%) had completed secondary school, 17 (10.2%) had completed secondary school and only 1 (0.6%) of the interviewees had higher education.

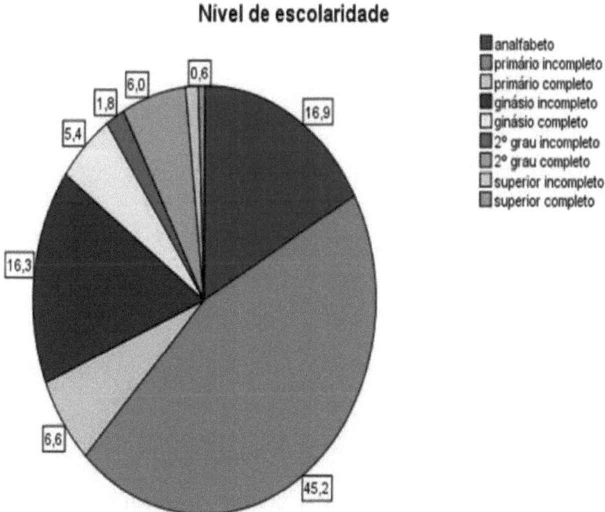

Figure 2 - Frequency of farmers in relation to ethnicity and location of study Source: Author of this dissertation, 2012.

When assessing working time in tobacco growing and with pesticides, the group had an average of 26.4±13.94 years and 42.25 ±15.99 hours per week (Table 3). Although the women worked on average longer (30 years) in tobacco growing than the men (23 years, p=0.006), the men continued to work more hours per week than the women (44 hours and 38 hours respectively, p=0.025).

Table 3 - Time spent working in tobacco growing using pesticides

Labour / Time	F	Mean ±SD	p-value
Years of Work	160	26,40 ±13,94	
Male	95	23,92 ±13,70	p=0,006
Female	65	30,03 ±13,57	
Hours/Week	154	42,25 ±15,99	
Male	92	44,62 ±14,68	p=0,025
Female	62	38,74 ±17,27	

Source: Author of this dissertation, 2012.

5.2 Symptomatic profile and lifestyle habits

A third of the 166 workers interviewed were smokers, i.e. 58 (34.9%), with no significant difference in terms of gender, and they consumed an average of 12 (± 9.96) cigarettes a day (Table 4).

Table 4 - Profile of rural workers who smoke

	Smoking	Non-smoker	p-value
Sex	58 (34,9%)	108 (65,1)	
Female	18 (26,9%)	49 (73,1%)	p=0,097
Male	40 (40,4%)	59 (59,6%)	
Cigarette consumption per day			
Mean ±SD:	12,61 ±9,96		
Frequency (%):			
<5 cigarettes/day	16 (28,1%)		
6 to 15 cigarettes/day	23 (40,4%)		
>16 cigarettes/day	18 (31,6%)		

Source: Author of this dissertation, 2012.

Regarding the prevalence of alcohol consumption among rural workers, 158 answered this question, indicating that 72 (45.6%) interviewees drank alcohol, with more men (61.2%) drinking alcohol than women (20%, p=0.001) (Table 5).

Table 5 - Prevalence of alcohol consumption among farmers in the rural community of Arapiraca (AL)

Sex	Alcoholic	Non-drinker	p-value
Female	12 (20%)	48 (80%)	p=0,001
Male	60 (61,2%)	38 (38,8%)	
Total	72 (45,6%)	86 (54,4%)	158

Source: Author of this dissertation, 2012.

Of the 158 interviewees who answered about the frequency of alcohol consumption, 58 (36.8%) drank up to three times a week, 31 (19.7%) drank four or more times a week, 17 (10.5%) drank once a week and 25 (15.7%) drank less than once a month (Figure 3).

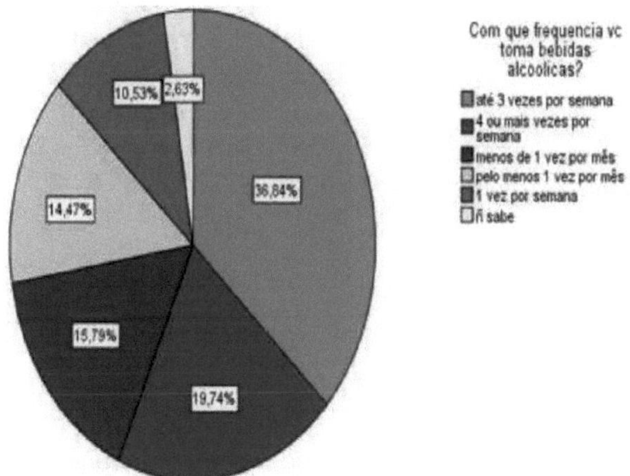

Figure 3 - Frequency of alcohol consumption by farmers Source: Author of this dissertation, 2012.

Considering the main complaints reported by 100 farmers, the data showed that headache (70%), nausea (45%), vomiting (42%) and vertigo (40%) were the most frequent symptoms, respectively (Table 6).

Table 6 - Most frequently reported symptoms among farmers

Symptoms*	F (%)
Nausea	45 (45,0%)
Headache	70 (70,0%)
Vomiting	42 (42,0%)
Vertigo	40 (40,0%)
Decreased vision	28 (28,0%)
Diarrhoea	19 (19,0%)
Chest pains	16 (16,0%)
Tremors	32 (32,0%)
Skin irritation	27 (27,0%)
Others	22 (22,0%)

*Each individual can have more than one symptom simultaneously.

Source: Author of this dissertation, 2012.

When assessing the presence of nicotinic symptoms (tremors) in farmers exposed to pesticides from the pyrethroid, neonicotinoid, strobilurin and organophosphate chemical groups, there was no significant difference between those who were symptomatic and those who were asymptomatic (p=0.626; 0.746; 0.204 and 0.962 respectively). The presence of muscarinic symptoms (nausea, vomiting, vertigo, diarrhoea and reduced vision) was also assessed, showing a significant difference only in individuals exposed to organophosphates with 26 (83.9%) cases compared to those not exposed in 34 (58.6%) cases (p=0.015) (Table 7).

Table 7 - Evaluation between exposure to organophosphates and reports of muscarinic symptoms in farmers

Organophosphates	Muscarinic Symptoms		Total	p-value
	Yes	No		
Exhibition	26 (83,9%)	5 (16,1%)	31	
Non-exposure	34 (58,6%)	24 (41,4%)	58	p=0,0 15
Total	60	29	89	

Source: Author of this dissertation, 2012. *Chi-squared test.

5.3Characterisation of tobacco farmers' occupational exposure to pesticides

According to the data obtained on the type of contact that tobacco farmers were exposed to pesticides, it was identified that the highest frequency was direct contact - through handling and applying the pesticide in 124 (79%) individuals. In these figures, it should be borne in mind that some of the farmers interviewed performed more than one function (Table 8).

Table 8 - Type of contact with pesticides that tobacco farmers were exposed to

Type of contact	F (%)
Direct Contact - handles and applies	124 (79)
Direct Contact - Pull the hose	9 (5,7)
Indirect contact - ploughing the same land as the house	10 (6,4)
Indirect contact - washes the costal	6 (3,8)
Indirect Contact - Washes clothes used in the application	13 (8,3)
Indirect Contact - is in the field during application	8 (5,1)
Contact other	5 (3,2)
Total	175 (111,5)

Source: Author of this dissertation, 2012.

Of the 166 individuals surveyed, 128 (81.5%) were directly exposed to pesticides - regardless of the type of direct contact. When assessed by gender, men were more likely to be in direct contact (90.8%) than women (66.1%), as shown in Table 9.

Table 9 - Type of contact with pesticides in relation to farmers' gender

Sex	Contact Direct	Contact Indirect	Tota	p-value

	F (%)	F (%)	- I	
Female	39 (66,1%)	20(33,9%)	59	0,001
Male	89 (90,8%)	9(9,2%)	98	
Total	128 (81,5%)	29(18,5%)	157	

Chi-squared test for p<0.05.

Source: Author of this dissertation, 2012.

When the chemical groups used in tobacco cultivation were analysed, pyrethroids with 108 (35.5%) had the highest frequency, followed by neonicotinoids with 80 (26.3%) and organophosphates with 40 (13.2%) (Table 10).

Table 10 - Chemical groups used in tobacco growing in Arapiraca (AL)

Chemical groups	F (%)	Cases
Pyrethroid	108 (35,5)	80,6%
Organophosphate	40 (13,2)	29,9%
Neonicotinoid	80 (26,3)	59,7%
Strobilurins	18 (5,9)	13,4%
Dimitroanilines	10 (3,3)	7,5%
Oxine methylcarbamate	8 (2,6)	6,0%
T riazole	7 (2,3)	5,2%
Carboxamide	4 (1,3)	3,0%
Bipyridylium	6 (2,0)	4,5%
Aryloxyphenoxypropionic acid	2 (0,7)	1,5%
Organotin	3 (1,0)	2,2%
Inorganic	5 (1,6)	3,7%
Dithiocarbamate	5 (1,6)	3,7%
Substituted glycine	3 (1,0)	2,2%
Aryloxyalkanoic Acid + Acid pyridinecarboxylic acid	3 (1,0)	2,2%
Fluoroaliphatic sulfonamides	1 (0,3)	0,7%
Naphthyl methylcarbamate	1 (0,3)	0,7%

Source: Author of this dissertation, 2012. *Each individual may have used more than one type of chemical group.

5.4 Characterisation of the blood count and serum biochemical profile of tobacco farmers exposed to pesticides

5.4.1 Socioeconomic, demographic and lifestyle variables

The results of haematological tests carried out on 166 rural workers who handled pesticides in tobacco growing in Arapiraca were analysed. The data was analysed in relation to age, gender, ethnicity and

of alcohol and tobacco consumption to identify possible variations associated with these characteristics. The individuals were grouped according to exposure characteristics, forming various subgroups.

In the gender comparison analyses, several items showed significant differences, as can be seen in Table 11. In the erythrogramme, the results showed higher values in males. The results of the leucogram (leucocytes, rods and lymphocytes) and platelets were higher in females. With the exception of globulins and phosphorus, all the other results were higher in males.

Table 11 - Evaluation between haematological test results with a significant difference and the gender of tobacco workers in Arapiraca (AL)

Tests	U	Reference Value	Female (F) Mean±SD a	Male(M) Mean ±SD	p-value
Haematocrit	%	F(36-47) M(40-54)	39,89 ±3,25	45,37 ±3,12	0,001
Haemoglobin	%	F(11,5-16) M(13,5-18)	13,18 ±116, i18	15,12 ±109,95	) 0,001
Red blood cells	%	4 - 5,6	4,59 ±0,34	5,15 ±0,41	0,001
VCM	%	80-100	86,54 ±54,94	88,01 ±38,47 0	0,053
HCM	%	27-32	28,56 ±22,94	29,25 ±17,47 0	0,039
CHCM	%	32-36	33,12 ±0,58	33,35 ±0,52	0,010
Leucocytes	MM^3	5000-1000(0	7.435 ±2.34 0	6.671 ±1.581	0,017
Sticks	MM^3	150-500	169.2 ±174, 6 00	117,5 ±87,39 9	) 0,016
Lymphocytes	MM3	103 -35 00	2.495 ±716, 48	2.053 ±535,4 8	t 0,000
Platelets	MM3	140.000 400.000	252.3 ±59.5 22 76	215.3 ±45.76 15 7	> 0,000
Urea	mg/d L	13-43	22,68 ±6,94	25,26 ±7,36	0,026
Uric acid	mg/d L	2,6-6	3,77 ±10,6 4	4,89 ±12,68	! 0,031
Albumin	g/dL	3,6-4,9	4,54 ±0,30	4,69 ±0,48	0,031
Globulin s	g/dL	1,9-3,1	3,24 ±0,54	3,01 ±0,69	0,032
A/G ratio	g/dL	1,4-2,3	1,44 ±0,30	1,66 ±0,48	0,002
Phosphorus	Ep/L	2,7-4,5	2,90 ±0,47	2,67 ±0,48	0,004
Sodium	Eq/L	138-145	143,8 ±2,26 8	145,8 ±2,31 0	0,001
Bilirubin a Direct	mg/d L	0,1-0,5	0,15 ±0,06	0,21±0,08	0,001
AST	UK/ mL	4,0-40	21,97 ±7,54	27,94 ±12,75	0,001
ALT	UK/ mL	4,0-36	20,59 ±7,88	27,41±12,18	0,001
Magnesium	Eq/L	1,6-2,4	2,00 ±0,19	2,14±0,39	0,013

Female (n=61), Male (n=92).

Source: Author of this dissertation, 2012.

Due to the possible interference that test results can suffer in relation to the individual's gender, many of which are confirmed in the literature, the analyses were separated according to this criterion.

Table 12 shows the significant biochemical and haematological results considering the age group of the individual, divided into up to forty years old and over forty years old. This criterion was defined based on the general average age of the individuals. Regardless of gender, individuals over 40 had higher glucose, total cholesterol, LDL cholesterol and lactate dehydrogenase values than younger individuals.

Women over forty showed significantly higher levels of liver transaminases than younger women. Only albumin levels in men up to the age of 40 were higher than the older group.

Table 12 - Serum biochemical results with a significant difference in relation to the age group up to 40 years and over 40 years of workers in Arapiraca (AL)

Tests	**Up to 40 years old**		**Over 40**		p-value
	Avera ge	**± SD**	**Mean ± SD**		
General		**(n=62)**	**(n=89)**		
Glucose	83,03	12,58	88,24	13,69	0,020
Cholesterol	178,73	44,85	202,98	39,64	0,001
LDL	113,39	42,35	128,64	32,16	0,013
LDH	321,12	61,10	364,77	77,96	0,001
Female (n=22)			**(n=39)**		
AST	18,79	3,43	23,788	,61	0,009
ALT	17,75	6,52	22,	218,19	0,026
Gender Male (n=40)			**(n=50)**		
Albumin	4,82	0,56	4,59	0,40	0,026

Source: Author of this dissertation, 2012. ***Student's t-test for p** á **0.05.**

When comparing the biochemical and haematological variables with the ethnicity of the farmers, it was only possible to observe differences when compared with the self-described black ethnic group. Table 13 shows the haematological variables with significant differences in relation to ethnicity.

Average triglyceride and GGT levels were higher in black individuals, regardless of their gender. Haematocrit and haemoglobin values were lower in black individuals, both female and male. In black women, the average albumin and phosphorus levels were lower than in mestizos and whites. In black men, the level of globulins was the highest (Table 13).

Table 13 - Evaluation of biochemical and haematological results of workers with a significant difference according to ethnicity

Tests	Black		Other Ethnicities		
	Average	±DP	Average	±DP	p-value
General	**(n=44)**		**(n=107)**		
Triglycerides	164,43	111,1	124,15	96,53	0,033
GGT	39,44	54,8	27,54	19,22	0,045
Female	**(n=21)**		**(n=40)**		
Haematocrit	38,62	3,44	40,55	2,98	0,026
Haemoglobin	12,64	1,22	13,46	1,03	0,008
CHCM	32,77	0,65	33,30	0,45	0,002
Albumin	4,42	0,35	4,59	0,26	0,036
Relationship A/G	1,34	0,24	1,50	0,33	0,050
Phosphorus	3,07	0,37	2,81	0,50	0,043
Male (n=23)			**(n=67)**		
Haematocrit	44,30	2,49	45,87	3,14	0,034
Haemoglobin	14,66	0,91	15,31	1,07	0,010
Sticks	155,91	113,50	103,60	72,63	0,048
Globulin s	3,51	0,76	2,82	0,58	0,001
Relationship A/G	1,44	0,57	1,75	0,42	0,007

Source: Author of this dissertation, 2012. ***Student's** t-test used **for p < 0.05.**

The variables that showed a significant difference between smokers and non-smokers are shown in Table 14. It can be seen that the levels of triglycerides, potassium and GGT were higher in the group of smokers. The haematological tests, which are interfered with by gender, showed no significant difference between the female subjects. In male smokers, the number of leucocytes was higher than non-smokers, but the urea level was lower than the other group.

Table 14 - Most significant haematological test results in relation to smoking prevalence in tobacco farmers

Tests	Smoker		Non-smoker		
	Average	± SD	Average	± SD	p-value
General	**(n=51)**		**(n=102)**		
Triglycerides	180,57	136,01	138,18	84,83	0,015
Potassium	4,85	0,37	4,70	0,40	0,034
GGT	45,93	71,09	30,44	26,61	0,049
Male (n=36)			**(n=56)**		
Leucocyte s	7.104	1.734	6.393	1.421	0,035
Urea	23,22	6,68	26,68	7,54	0,022

Source: Author of this dissertation, 2012. ***Student's t-test for p <** 0.05.

When the workers were grouped according to alcohol consumption, the alcoholics had higher values for total cholesterol, triglycerides and GGT (Table 15).

The mean values for the following variables: urea, uric acid and phosphorus were higher in women who drank alcohol than in women who didn't drink alcohol. Sodium was lower in women who drank alcohol. Men who were alcoholics had higher levels of uric acid and sodium than non-alcoholics. Only ALT transaminase was lower in male alcoholics.

Table 15 - Significant serum biochemical results in relation to the prevalence of alcoholic tobacco workers in Arapiraca (AL)

Tests	Alcoholic		Non-drinker		Value of p
	Average	± SD	Average	± SD	
General	(n=63)		(n=83)		
Cholesterol	200,46	44,98	185,92	42,23	0,039
Triglycerides	177,28	128,99	134,27	85,53	0,014
GGT	45,71	50,82	29,35	45,84	0,038
Female	(n=10)		(n=45)		
Urea	26,66	6,82	21,74	6,99	0,033
Uric Acid	4,31	1,21	3,56	0,96	0,025
Phosphorus	3,15	0,58	2,84	0,44	0,058
Sodium	142,25	2,37	144,44	1,80	0,007
Male	(n=53)		(n=38)		
Uric acid	5,09	1,25	4,55	1,24	0,043
Sodium	146,45	2,35	144,50	1,64	0,027
ALT	25,43	9,89	30,37	14,86	0,054

Source: Author of this dissertation, 2012. *Student's t-test for $p < 0.05$.

With regard to the possible interference of the use of medication, it was identified that of the 166 individuals in the sample, 105 used some kind of medication. Of these, 9 (5.4%) used medication indicated for hypertension, 3 (1.8%) for heart problems and 6 (3.6%) for neurological diseases, which are chronic medications, and 28 (16.8%) for other medications. It was not possible to carry out statistical analyses, given that there were few individuals identified as using medication for each subgroup.

5.4.2 . Evaluation of exposure to pesticides

The variables collected were analysed in relation to exposure to individual groups of pesticides. In this case, workers were grouped according to their exposure to the four main chemical groups used: pyrethroids, organophosphates, neonicotinoids and strobilurins.

Table 16 shows the relationship between haematological and biochemical tests in relation to exposure to pyrethroid pesticides. It can be seen that potassium levels are high in individuals exposed to the pesticide. Women exposed to pyrethroids had lower erythrocyte indices (haematocrit, haemoglobin and number of red blood cells) than those not exposed to this pesticide. Urea and phosphorus levels were higher among exposed women and ALT transaminase was lower, also among those exposed. In exposed men, uric acid levels were lower than in unexposed men.

Table 16 - Results of significant haematological tests and the use of pyrethroid pesticides in tobacco growing

Tests	Pyrethroid pesticide				p-value
	Exposed		Non-Exposed		
	n	Mean±SD	n	Mean±SD	
GENERAL					
Potassium	73	4,8±0,4	23	4,6±0,3	0,030
FEMALE					
Haematocrit	27	39,2 ±2,7	14	42,0 ±3,2	0,007
Haemoglobin	27	12,9 ±0,9	14	13,9 ±1,0	0,009
Red blood cells	27	4,55 ±0,3	14	4,79 ±0,3	0,053
Urea	30	24,73 ±6,9	15	19,40 ±5,2	0,012
ALT	31	17,64 ±5,4	15	22,7 ±8,0	0,015
Phosphorus	29	3,04 ±0,3	14	2,58 ±04	0,001
MALE SEX					
Uric Acid	76	4,71 ±1,2	11	5,54 ±1,3	0,044

Source: Author of this dissertation, 2012. Student's t-test for p á 0.05.

The exposure of tobacco workers to organophosphates and the significance of the tests can be seen in Table 17. Men exposed to this chemical group had higher platelet levels. In addition, exposed individuals had higher HDL and lower lipase values than non-exposed individuals. However, only men under 40 showed a reduction in lipase levels.

Table 17 - Results of significant haematological tests and the use of organophosphate pesticides in tobacco growing

Tests	Organophosphate pesticide				p-value
	Exposed		Non-Exposed		
	n	Mean±SD	n	Mean±SD	
GENERAL					
HDL	40	44,1 ±10,2	90	40,5 ±8,8	0,041
Lipase	29	31,6 ±7,6	68	36,6 ±11,4	0,031
MALE SEX					
Platelets	23	236.174 ±44.418	58	209.638 ±45.336	0,019

Source: Author of this dissertation, 2012. **Student's t-test for p** á 0.05.

When comparing the average lipase levels in relation to the working time of exposed individuals, separated by groups, it was possible to observe that individuals with up to ten years of work had lower lipase levels (26.4) than those over thirty years

(35.4; $p<0.05$) (Figure 4). When the correlation between working time and lipase levels in exposed individuals was assessed, there was significance (0.028) indicating a weak ($r=0.359$) but positive correlation, where lipase increases with working time for both genders, as seen in Figure 4.

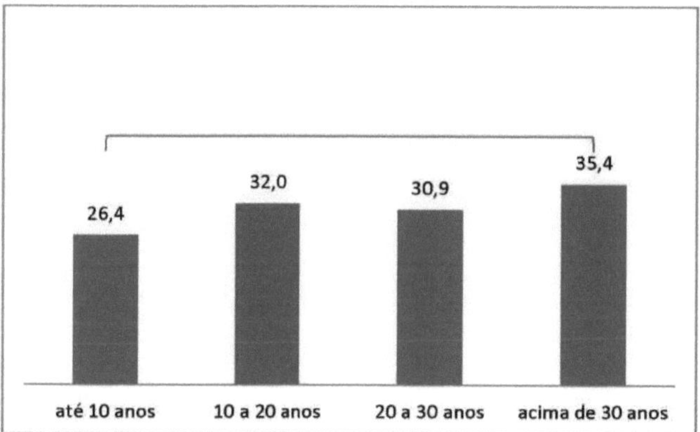

Figure 4 - Average lipase levels in relation to working time of individuals exposed to organophosphates separated by groups

Source: Author of this dissertation, 2012. Pearson's chi-square for p á 0.05

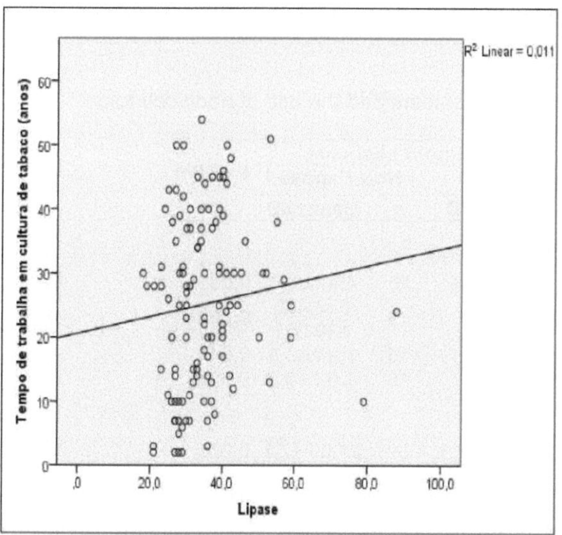

Figure 5 - Correlation between working time and lipase levels in individuals exposed to organophosphates

zSource: Author of this dissertation, 2012. Correlation p=0.028;

r=0,359.

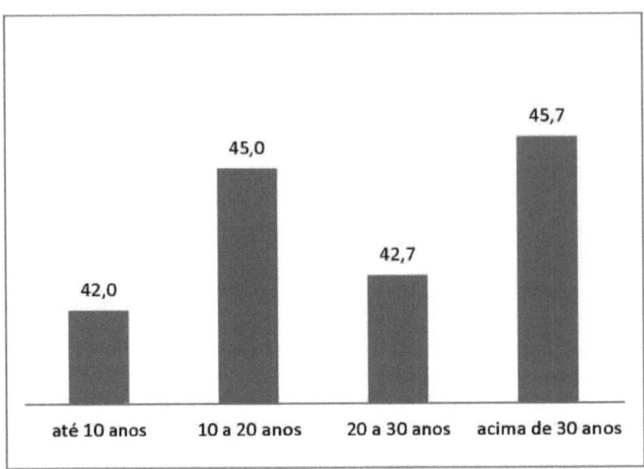

Figure 6 - Average HDL levels in relation to working hours of individuals exposed to organophosphates, separated by group.

Source: Author of this dissertation, 2012. Test of

ANOVA (p>0.05).

When exposed to neonicotinoid pesticides, women showed higher results in terms of red blood cells, platelets, as well as globulin and magnesium levels than women not exposed to this pesticide (Table 18). Among exposed men, only urea levels were significantly lower than non-exposed men.

Table 18 - Results of significant haematological tests and the use of neonicotinoid pesticides in tobacco growing

Tests	Neonicotinoid pesticide				p-value
	Exposed		Non-Exposed		
	n	Mean±SD	n	Mean±SD	
FEMALE					
Red blood cells	26	4,73 ±0,3	15	4,47 ±0,4	0,035
Platelets	25	271.240 ±59.132	15	223.466 ±39.951	0,009
Globulins	28	3,31 ±0,5	15	2,94 ±0,5	0,041
Magnesium	25	2,06 ±0,2	15	1,93 ±0,2	0,053
MALE SEX					
Urea	47	23,59 ±7,1	39	27,00 ±7,7	0,038

Source: Author of this dissertation, 2012. Student's t-test **for p 0.05.**

As for exposure to pesticides in the strobilurin group, the significant tests are shown in Table 19. Regardless of gender, LDH and GGT levels were elevated in individuals exposed to strobilurins. No comparison was made between women, as only one was exposed to this pesticide. Among the results observed in males, the number of lymphocytes, globulin levels, phosphorus and magnesium were lower in the group exposed to the pesticide. The A/G ratio was higher in those exposed than those not exposed to the strobilurin.

Table 19 - Results of significant haematological tests and the use of strobilurin pesticides in tobacco growing

Tests	Strobilurin pesticide				p-value
	Exposed		Non-Exposed		
	n	Mean±SD	n	Mean±SD	
GENERAL					
LDH	18	380,61 ±74,3	111	336,36 ±72,6	0,018
GGT	18	45,16 ±36,0	112	29,49 ±22,4	0,014
MALE SEX					
Lymphocytes	17	1.830 ±674	64	2.119 ±479	0,047
Globulins	17	2,38 ±0,5	67	3,12 ±0,6	0,001
Magnesium	16	1,98 ±0,3	55	2,20 ±0,4	0,050

Source: Author of this dissertation, 2012. **Student's t-test for $p < 0.05$.**

CHAPTER 6

DISCUSSION

The Ministry of Health in its Guidelines for Comprehensive Health Care for Workers of Differentiated Complexity in the Protocol for Health Care for Workers Exposed to Pesticides suggests that complementary tests should be carried out, such as a full blood count, total proteins and fractions, total bilirubin and fractions, alkaline phosphatase, AST, ALT urea, creatinine and others (SILVA et al., 2006). However, it does not specify their importance as possible biomarkers for intoxication and does not provide analysis parameters for health professionals to conduct investigations into this type of exposure. From this perspective, it is extremely important to develop research to subsidise the health assessment carried out in healthcare.

This study sought to characterise the blood count and serum biochemical profile of individuals exposed to pesticides in the Arapiraca (AL) tobacco industry. Its purpose was to evaluate the effects of exposure and to subsidise future research into the health-disease process of pesticide applicators, as well as the chronic effects of these compounds on the population.

6.1 Socio-economic, demographic and occupational profiles of tobacco workers

The profile of exposure to pesticides among tobacco workers showed that the group studied had an average of 26 years of work with a significant working week of forty-two hours, which had been repeated since adolescence. According to Baldi et al. (2003), this exposure increases the risk of lower cognitive performance with each additional year and of developing Alzheimer's or Parkinson's disease in men.

Almost 60 per cent of the population studied were men and they were exposed to high quantities of pesticides, as well as handling and applying them, which increases the risk of poisoning (FILLA & VESTENA, 2008) and diseases associated with this type of contact. According to Nascimento and Silva (2011), women start working in tobacco growing earlier, using plastic containers to apply the pesticide. In fact, this type of application is characteristic of women tobacco growers, who apply the product from below, close to the root, and run the risk of being bitten by a snake, for example.

Although in our study the women reported working fewer hours a week in the cultivation area, they start working as applicators from a young age and are exposed to the aggression produced by this product earlier in their development. They also live close to the planting area, which increases their exposure. Men, on the other hand, start working with tobacco later, in activities that require more strength.

During the application of agrochemicals to crops using a backpack pump, the agrochemicals usually overflow and run down the applicator's back. The malfunctioning of these devices is another concern, since they are practically maintenance-free and usually have defects such as clogged pumps and a lack of adequate pressure to propel the liquid, which means that the farmer's hands get wet throughout the application. In addition to this, the lack of use of PPE by farmers in Arapiraca (AL) (NASCIMENTO, 2011) is another aggravating factor for the health of tobacco workers.

Among the socio-economic aspects, the low level of schooling identified in this population was worrying. The survey revealed that almost half of the sample (75) had less than four years of schooling, a factor that contributes to increasing the impact of human contamination by pesticides (OLIVEIRA-SILVA, 2001), as it is a limiting factor for the ability to read and interpret the labels of the products used by farmers (PERES, 2003; SOARES et al., 2005). Difficulty in reading instructions on pesticide dilution and the grace period (the interval between one application of the product and another) are some of the situations that increase the risk of farmers falling ill.

The illiteracy rate presented in this study was one sixth of the sample 28 (16.9%). When compared to the national rate, it was almost twice as high as that identified for Brazil in the 2010 census (FUNDAÇÃO INSTITUTO BRASILEIRO DE GEOGRAFIA E ESTATÍSTICA, 2010). This reflects the greater vulnerability of this population to poisoning compared to other regions of the country and reinforces the statement by the Department of Rural Socioeconomic Studies (2008) about the lack of preparation for working in tobacco growing.

For the classification of ethnic groups in this research, we used the same criteria as the national study by Bydlowski et al. (2001) and the one adopted by the IBGE in carrying out the population census (METHODOLOGY OF THE DEMOGRAPHIC CENSUS, 2000, 2003) where individuals classify themselves as white, mixed race, black and Indian.

In this context, half of the workers called themselves mestizos, in line with the characteristics of the Brazilian population (METODOLOGIA DO CENSO DEMOGRÁFICO, 2010) and a third called themselves black. This number of black individuals was due to one of the locations **surveyed (Pau D'arco)** being predominantly quilombola, which justifies the difference in relation to Silva's study (2011) where the majority were mixed race and white. This variable was not considered in several studies (ARCURY et al., 2001; LEVIRGAD, 2001; BEDOR, 2008; NASCIMENTO, 2011). However, it is of paramount importance in susceptibility studies and for health assessments in different ethnic groups.

6.2 Symptomatic and lifestyle profiles

In our study, smoking was present in approximately a third of the sample (34.9%). In this population, 31.6% smoked more than sixteen cigarettes a day, which is worrying because it exposes these workers even more to pesticides, considering that they smoked during the application and handling of these products (SILVA, 2011). In the study by Faria et al. (2009), few rural workers reported smoking and, among those who did smoke, cigarette consumption per day was lower than in our study.

Contact with pesticides can make farmers ill. The toxicity of these substances occurs through various mechanisms of action. Junior et al. (1999) report that when nicotinic and central nervous system receptors are excited by pesticides, the stimuli can cause important signs and symptoms such as tachycardia, hypertension and alterations in electrocardiogram (EEG) results.

Associated with smoking, these physiological changes can be aggravated due to the increase in blood pressure (BP). Rocha et al. (1998) mention that blood pressure can be raised by smoking cigarettes, which increases blood flow to the heart, helping to increase cardiac output (CONTRAN et al., 2000; BATISTA et al., 2009; ARAÚJO, 2009). These alterations, when sufficient to overcome the body's efforts to keep functioning, can contribute to strokes in this population.

The prevalence of alcoholism among the participants in this study was similar to that of non-alcoholics, i.e. around fifty per cent, which is different to what Araújo et al. (2007) reported. We also found that one fifth (19.7 per cent) of the interviewees answered that they used alcohol four or more times a week, which coincides with Araújo et al. (2007).

It is common for farmers to drink alcohol at the end of their work (field work), but the quantity and number of times they do so is worrying. Alcohol is metabolised in the liver, which is also where the body's detoxification process takes place.

Damage to this important organ makes it impossible or limits the process of eliminating toxic substances such as pesticides, as well as modifying the behaviour of certain enzymes such as AST, ALT and GGT. Changes in the profile of these enzymes are relevant biomarkers for alcoholic interference. Chronic alcohol use interferes with GGT levels, where an isolated increase is associated with high alcohol consumption (CARVALHO et al., 2006) and a concomitant AST/ALT ratio greater than 2 is indicative of alcoholic aetiology (GONÇALVES et al., 2006).

Continued exposure to pesticides combined with alcohol consumption increases this population's risk of becoming ill. Furthermore, according to Almeida & Martins (2008), alcohol consumption is a confounding factor when assessing chronic pesticide poisoning, due to symptoms such as peripheral polyneuropathy and myopathy (SCHAUMBURG & BERGER, 1993; JAMAL, 1995).

The main symptoms of poisoning reported were nausea, vertigo, vomiting and headache. Similar to our study, these symptoms of the peripheral nervous system (muscarinic) and central nervous system were also mentioned in other studies that reported that they resulted from contact with organophosphates (HEEMANN, 2009;

ROTHLEIN et al.; RECENA et al., 2006; SILVA, 2011; JENSEN et al., 2011).

The signs and symptoms they produce can be due to stimulation of muscarinic receptors (bradycardia, hypotension, sialorrhoea, nausea, vomiting, abdominal pain, diarrhoea, faecal incontinence, tenesmus, wheezing, miosis, lacrimation), nicotinic receptors (fasciculations, muscle weakness, paralysis, tachycardia, hypertension, mydriasis, sweating) or even causing changes in the central nervous system (altered consciousness, coma, convulsions, respiratory depression, Cheyne-Stoke breathing, ataxia, tremor, dysarthria) (JUNIOR et al., 1999; ORTIZ et al., 2009; RASTOGI, 2010).When relating pesticides to the symptoms reported by farmers, the data revealed that individuals exposed to organophosphates showed a significant difference in relation to muscarinic symptoms. This result is consistent with data in the literature showing that these insecticides can cause intoxication due to their anticholinesterase effect in mammals.

In addition, with chronic exposure, individuals can develop depression, which is a determining factor in cases of suicide. Diagnoses of late-onset neuropathy, neurobehavioural syndrome and neuropsychiatric disorders have been linked to the chronic use of organophosphates (ARAÚJO et al., 2007). However, these parameters were not assessed in the sample.

6.3 Characterisation of tobacco farmers' occupational exposure to pesticides

The level of exposure to pesticides was characterised based on the chemical groups used and the type of contact, in line with reports in various studies (SOARES et al.; FEHLBERG et al., 2003; SOUSA et al., 2011; JENSEN et al., 2011). The greater the exposure, the greater the risk over time of falling ill (MOREIRA et al., 2002), with neurological diseases, rheumatoid arthritis (MILHAM, 1988; OLSSON, 2004) and oral diseases, as well as being twice as likely to report pain (SOUZA et al., 2011).

Our population consisted of applicators, but some of them did more than one job, which meant more hours on the farm and consequently greater exposure to the pesticides dispersed. Predominantly, the pesticides were of toxicological class II (moderately toxic), IV (very slightly toxic) and I (highly toxic), respectively. The most commonly used pesticides were Deltamethine (Decis), Imidacloprid (Confidor), Lambda-Cyhalothrin (Karate), Methamidophos (Tamaron) and Azoxystrobin (Amistar), respectively.

With regard to the chemical category, the pesticides most used in tobacco growing were pyrethroids, neonicotinoids and organophosphates, respectively. This result is in line with that reported by Nascimento (2011). Research carried out in Pernambuco and other countries, such as Cambodia and Pakistan, found that organophosphates and pyrethroids were among the most cited (SALEEM, 2008; BEDOR et al., 2007; LATORRACA et al., 2008; BEDOR, 2009; JENSEN et al., 2011).

According to Macário (2007), among the pesticides in use, organophosphates are responsible for most cases of acute and chronic poisoning. (2002) the threshold for neurotoxic consequences, commonly related to high doses of OFs, can be exacerbated during repeated exposure to low doses of this chemical, even when the agents are considered moderately toxic or non-neuropathic, such as chlorpyrifos (CPF).

6.4 Characterisation of the blood count and serum biochemical profile of tobacco farmers

Health assessment requires biomarkers as one of its components. The biomonitoring of exposure to pesticides is important because it serves as a biological parameter of exposure (AMORIM et al., 2003). These instruments are effective in helping to make decisions regarding the prevention of the effects caused by pesticides (BERLIN et al., 1982). Depending on their magnitude, biomarkers of effect can signal a health problem or even a pre-established disease (BRASIL, 2004).

(2003), establishing a relationship between exposure and the effects produced on the health of individuals is of paramount importance in order to better estimate the risk. Monitoring the haematological parameters of farmers can be useful for preventing health risks caused by pesticides (ABU et al., 2005; ARAOUD et al., 2012).

The assessment of enzymatic activity has been very useful as a bioindicator and has shown that excessive exposure has its own clinical or toxicological significance, which may be associated with an effect or dysfunction of the biological system being assessed (AZEVEDO; CHASIN, 2003).

To assess the haematological parameters of tobacco farmers exposed to pesticides, gender-dependent interferences were considered, in agreement with Baldi et al. (2003). For Stopelli & Magalhães (2005), variations in gender, age, ethnicity, nutritional status, smoking and drinking habits, ethnicity and genetics should also be taken into account.

VCM and HCM levels comparing both sexes ($p = 0.053$; $p = 0.039$) resulted in higher values for men in the reference value range. Hernández et al. (2005) and Araoud et al. (2012) believe that analysing these variables is extremely important for biomonitoring, as variations, even subtle ones, can guide investigations into exposure to pesticides. Caldas et al. (2000) reinforce this statement when they suggest that these tests should be carried out when investigating poisoning.

Serum biochemical levels of aspartate aminotransferase (AST), alanine aminotransferase (ALT) and gamma glutamyl transferase (GGT) were analysed in this study using different groupings. When the reference values for AST (4 - 40) and ALT (4 - 36) were analysed, it was noted that the aminotransferase levels in women showed averages closer to the minimum threshold, lower than those in men, as confirmed by the literature (DUFOUR, 2000).

Some authors have reported a relationship between the altered activity of these enzymes in toxicity assessments of workers exposed to organophosphates or in combination with other pesticides (ANWAR, 1997; KHAN et al., 2008). Araoud et al. (2012) correlated the number of years of exposure to pesticides with higher ALT activity. These enzymes generally increase their activity in patients with liver disease and can be considered a specific marker of liver damage (PRATT, 1990).

When comparing the GGT results with the reference values (1-38), the dosages of black individuals and alcoholics were above the limit value. Parron et al. (1996) also reported an increase in GGT due to contact with pesticides. In the study by Nunez et al. (1998) there was an increase in GGT when comparing the activities of this enzyme before and after spraying, although not significant and within normal values, they do not exclude the possible presence of disease.

This study analysed inorganic substances such as calcium, potassium, phosphorus and sodium. Phosphorus levels were higher in black women and alcoholics. Parron et al. (1996) also reported an increase in inorganic phosphorus in 7% of the cohort of pesticide sprayers.

With regard to age, the mean levels of glucose, cholesterol, LDL-c and LDH were higher for both genders aged over forty.

Considering that this population was exposed to pesticides, that this is a form of injury to the body, and that the biochemical variables cholesterol, LDL-c and LDH are predictors of heart disease (SILVA & MARQUES, 2007; MONTEIRO, 2011), it can be considered that their increase with age increases the risk of cardiovascular disease.

The smokers were grouped according to their smoking habits. This group of smokers and non-smokers was assessed considering the characteristics of the blood count and serum biochemical profile of this subgroup.

An increase in triglyceride (0.015), potassium (0.034) and GGT (p=0.049) levels was observed in smokers, which was significant when compared to non-smokers. Similarly, Prigol et al. (2007), when considering the lipid profile of smokers, identified that from the consumption of twenty cigarettes a day, this habit directly interferes with the dosages of cholesterol, LDL-c and triglycerides, increasing them in relation to control groups and significantly decreasing HDL-c (GUEDES et al., 2007).

Robinson and Whitehead (1989) found in men a gradual increase in GGT between groups and the number of cigarettes per day. Several other studies have reported that smoking has a significant effect on the increase in GGT (WANNAMETHEE et al., 1995; WHITEHEAD et al., 1996; JOUSILAHTI et al., 2000). In our study, male smokers showed an increase in the number of leucocytes and a decrease in urea levels. Similarly, Carvalho et al. (2008) identified that tobacco consumption can promote an increase in the number of leucocytes.

Studies have shown that the liver is a primary target organ in cases of acute and chronic exposure to pesticides, and therefore alterations in liver function would be more sensitive indicators of toxic reactions induced by these substances (NUNEZ et al., 1998). According to these authors, one of the most common laboratory alterations among rural workers exposed to pesticides is the GGT enzyme, as already mentioned in the text. According to Walter et al. (1990) its increase can be due to hepatobiliary disease, alcoholism, acute and chronic pancreatitis and prostate adenocarcinoma.

6.5 Evaluation of haematological and serum biochemical changes in tobacco farmers

The data was stratified according to the exposure of individuals to the most commonly used chemical groups (organophosphates, pyrethroids, neonicotinoids and strobilirorins), with the aim of identifying physiological changes resulting from contact with a specific class of pesticides. In this case, exposed and unexposed subgroups were separated for each chemical group, which allowed us to identify variations potentially related to these compounds.

6.5.1 Organophosphates

Organophosphate class pesticides are commonly used in agriculture (FORGET, 1991; ASPERLIN, 1994) and have been the most widely used in the world since the 1970s (BARTH & BIAZON, 2010). In 1999, OFs accounted for 40 per cent of the world market (SANTOS et al., 2007) and today they are still one of the three most widely used pesticides in Brazil (BEDOR, 2008). These chemicals cause alterations in some haematological and biochemical parameters in experimental animals and humans (KAZMI et al., 2003; JACOBSON et al., 2004).

Considering the individuals exposed to organophosphates in relation to those who do not use this pesticide, a significant difference was identified in the values for pancreatic lipase and HDL. However, the values for lipase were reduced ($p = 0.031$) and HDL was increased ($p = 0.041$) when compared to the non-exposed group. The difference in lipase levels was only observed in the under-40 group. In this respect, we also described a positive correlation between increasing age or working hours and lipase levels, only in the exposed group.

According to Caside et al. (2008), organophosphates can inhibit lipases, e.g. monoacylglycerol, which modulate the levels of enzymes in the brain that are linked to pain, motility and memory processes. The author considers that the various lipid systems in the brain are modulated by lipases that are highly sensitive to these pesticides.

For Terry (2012), the high reactivity of OFs can alter the function of other enzymes and proteins, in addition to cholinesterase. He also suggests that long-term exposure can affect some basic neuronal processes, as has been associated with neuropsychiatric symptoms.

Experimental data shows that OFs cause a functional obstruction of the pancreatic ducts, at the same time as they stimulate pancreatic exocrine secretions, so there is interstitial oedema in the pancreas, vacuolisation in the acinar cells, resulting in hyperamylasemia and hyperlipasemia (DRESSEL et al., 1979). Cholinergic hyperstimulation of the pancreatic acinar cell can cause an increase in lipase due to acute pancreatitis (FRICK et al., 1987). According to Caldas (2000), individuals occupationally exposed to organophosphates may have pancreatic lipase levels three or more times higher than normal, resulting in some cases of pancreatitis. Carboxyl esterases, known as lipases, catalyse the hydrolysis of triacylglycerols with long aliphatic chains (VERGER, 1997; SHARMA et al., 2001).

The decrease in lipase observed in the OF-exposed group, compared to the non-exposed group, may indicate a reduction in the activity of this enzyme in the body, as assessed by the enzymatic test. On the other hand, the increase in lipase levels over time may suggest a compromised pancreas due to chronic exposure to OF. These two mechanisms could be counterbalancing the levels of this enzyme so that in the group over 40 years of age no difference was detected in relation to unexposed individuals. It is possible that other lipases in the body are also influenced by exposure to OF, which may be related to the cases of intoxication reported in the literature. Further studies may indicate whether pancreatic lipase is a good biomarker of exposure to these compounds.

There is some evidence that cholinergic stimulation by sufficiently high exposure to organophosphates promotes cell proliferation, which represents the possible development of tumours, for example mammary tumours (CABELLO et al., 2001).

In our study, the men exposed to OFs had higher platelet counts than the group not exposed to these pesticides ($p = 0.019$).

Rasgoti et al. (2012) showed that exposure to pesticides significantly decreased the average platelet count when comparing the exposed group (sprayers) with the control group ($p < 0.05$). However, Abu et al. (2005) when assessing the impact of exposure to organophosphates on Palestinians in the Gaza Strip, identified an increase in the amount of platelets after spraying, reflecting acute intoxication.

Our findings are similar to those found by Abu et al. in that we evaluated the effect of exposure to these chemical compounds compared to other applicators and not to a group not exposed to pesticides. We cannot say at this stage whether the platelet levels of the study population are higher or lower than those of the unexposed control group.

6.5.2 Pyrethroids

In this study, the group of women exposed to pyrethroids had haematocrit, haemoglobin and red blood cells with averages close to the minimum threshold when compared to reference values and lower levels when compared to the non-exposed group ($p = 0.007$; $p = 0.009$; $p = 0.053$, respectively).

This pattern was also observed when these markers were analysed with the confounding variables, which showed that they were variations resulting from the influence of pyrethroid use. The reduction in these levels was in line with the results of Patil et al (2003). According to these authors, exposure to pesticides can negatively influence the biosynthesis of the Heme group and, as a consequence, the production of haemoglobin and red blood cells, influencing the reduction in haematocrit.

In addition, studies carried out on rats treated orally with low and high concentrations of pyrethroids found changes in the physicochemical properties of the erythrocyte bilayer and changes in the activity of antioxidant enzymes (NASUTI et al., 2003), influencing haemolysis (Carneiro et al., 2007).

Pesticides are nephrotoxic to humans and can cause acute renal failure (COSTA, 1998). (SHAFEY et al., 2011). In this respect, serum values of urea, uric acid and creatinine, combined with other factors, can elucidate kidney damage processes (SODRÉ et al., 2007; BARTH & BIAZON, 2010).

In our study, women exposed to pyrethroids had higher urea levels than those not exposed. Similarly, results by Shafey et al. (2011) showed significantly increased plasma urea ($p < 0.05$) compared to controls, indicating damage to kidney cells or even kidney failure, since these changes can indicate kidney dysfunction characterised by reduced renal flow with a higher concentration of urea in the serum. Although we didn't compare our sample with controls, we don't rule out the possibility that the difference in our findings could be indicative of kidney cell damage.

In the study by Oliveira et al. (2011), workers exposed to pesticides maintained normal urea levels. Hernández et al. (2006) and Araoud et al. (2012) disagreed on the urea dosage, but both described that these analyses should be deepened in the health assessment of workers exposed to pesticides.

6.5.3 Neonicotinoids

When urea levels were analysed in relation to pesticides, there was significance in the relationships made with neonicotinoids, where men exposed to these substances had lower dosages than those not exposed, showing significant differences between the groups assessed.

In this study, magnesium levels were higher in exposed women than in unexposed women (p=0.053), showing significance, albeit at the limit. When the interfering covariates were analysed, it was only in alcoholics that this finding was reversed. This is consistent with the literature, in which an increase in alcohol concentration influences a decrease in serum magnesium (PETROIANU et al., 2004). Our findings were not significant, indicating that alcohol did not interfere with the increase in magnesium among the group exposed to neonicotinoids.

In addition, red blood cells, platelets, globulins and magnesium varied in females. To our knowledge, there is no data in the literature on the effect of this pesticide on the parameters analysed.

6.5.4 *Strobilurins*

The mean LDH (p = 0.018) and GGT (p = 0.014) of individuals exposed to strobilurins were higher than those not exposed in both sexes. An increase in these enzymes in serum can indicate damage to the liver or other tissues (KHAN et al., 2008). As the increase profile was similar for all the subgroups of interference variables tested, the effect observed may in fact be due to the action of this compound.

The lymphocyte count was also significant (p = 0.047) in males, where the average for those exposed was lower than for those not exposed. Although there are no studies on the effects of strobilurins on haematological data, there are studies on pesticide exposure where lymphopenia was one of the main findings (Meyer et al., 2003).

6.6 Final considerations

Although workers are constantly exposed to various pesticides, studies on the consequences of these exposures on human health are still insufficient. The simultaneous effects of using several pesticides at the same time are still unknown (QUANDT et al., 2004). In this respect, biomarkers could be used to indicate the adverse effects of pesticides on agricultural workers (ARAOUD et al., 2012).

It is important to emphasise that many pesticides have long-lasting effects on the body, even after the use of the agent has been discontinued. This is due to the long half-life, the persistence of active metabolites and the high liposolubility of many pesticides, leading them to be deposited in adipose tissue (SOUZA et al., 2011).

According to Yonamine (2005), in chronic pesticide poisoning, the clinical picture is undefined and the diagnosis difficult to establish. According to Faria et al.

(2007) it is difficult to characterise the exposure itself, largely due to the difficulty of obtaining information on the chronic effect, the lack of knowledge of health professionals in diagnosing and investigating, and the fact that many alterations do not trigger symptoms (ALMEIDA & MARTINS, 2008).

In general, although not significant in some cases, the mean values showed the same upward or downward trend in relation to exposure, regardless of the interference factor considered. When the values deviated from the trend, they were also not significant, with the exception of globulin in the female smoker group exposed to neonicotinoids. This lack of significance can be explained by the small number of individuals in some groups after stratification. For example, only 1 alcoholic was not exposed to neonicotinoids, which may have been responsible for the difference in the profiles observed in relation to the others.

In this way, the data indicate that the differences observed stem from the action of the compounds on the exposed workers' bodies and not from the effect of these variables. A covariate to be considered is the possible interference of alcoholism in the urea levels detected during exposure to neonicotinoids. Only the group exposed to alcohol showed a significant decrease in urea values, while the non-alcoholic group was the only one with a trend different from the rest, although not significant.

This study found that exposure to pesticides is associated with variations in various physiological parameters, suggesting that they may be due to the adverse effects of these substances on rural workers. In addition, various clinical symptoms related to intoxication were observed in the study population and, particularly in the group exposed to OFs, a prevalence of symptoms associated with muscarinic receptors, which have been shown to be interfered with by this compound. These observations reinforce the importance of routine biomonitoring to screen for possible effects on workers' health.

CHAPTER 7

CONCLUSIONS

The educational profile of the sample of tobacco growers investigated shows a low level of schooling, a factor that contributes to a greater risk of poisoning; many years of work in the same crop and in the same occupational activities. In addition, most of the tobacco growers have direct contact with pesticides and live in the same area of cultivation, contributing to a greater degree of exposure.

The main pesticides used on the crop were pyrethroids, neonicotinoids, organophosphates and strobilurins.

Various symptoms associated with pesticide poisoning have been reported. With regard to individuals exposed to OFs, a prevalence of muscarinic symptoms has been observed.

When analysing the effect of exposure to specific pesticides, significant differences were identified in various haematological and serum biochemical parameters, suggesting that these pesticides interfere with the physiology of the individuals.

Although there are not many reports in the literature on the chronic effect of exposure to pesticides, some of the alterations found are consistent with the action of these compounds, described in other studies.

The variations reported, although within normal limits, can in the long term contribute to the onset of serious pathologies such as neuropsychiatric disorders, cancer, pancreatic, hepatic and renal dysfunctions, among others.

The data suggest that periodic biological monitoring of exposed workers may be relevant for the early identification of potential physiological variations that cause these pathologies.

REFERENCES

ABU, M. T. Adverse impact of insecticides on the health of Palestinian farm workers in the Gaza Strip: a haematologic biomarker study. **Int J Occup Environ Health**, Crete, v. 11, n. 2, p. 144-149, 2005.

AITIO, A.; KALLIO, A. Exposure and effect monitoring: a critical appraisal of their practical application. **Toxicology Letters**, Finland, p.137-147, 1999.

AITIO, A. Biological monitoring today and tomorrow. **Scan. J. Environ. Health**, Helsinki, p. 46-58, 1994.

ALAVANJA, M. C. R., HOPPIN J. A.; KAMEL, F. Health effects of chronic pesticide exposure: cancer and neurotoxity. **Annu. Rev. Public Health**, North Carolina, p. 157-197, 2004.

ALMEIDA, G. E. G. Smoking: Modern Servitude and Violation of Human Rights. Land of Rights. Curitiba. 2005 . p. 168

ANDRADE, F. A.; CAMPOLINA, D.; DIAS,M. B. **Toxicologia na Prática Clínica.** 2. ed. Belo Horizonte: Folium, 2001.

ANWAR, W.A. Biomarkers of Human Exposure to Pesticides. **Environmental Health Perspective**, Cairo, v. 105, p. 801-806, 1997.

ARAOUD, M.; FADOUA, N.; WAHIBA, D.. HASSEN, B. H.; MOHAMED, A.; MOHSSEN, H.; MOHAMED, F. N.; ABDERRAOUF, K. Adverse effects of pesticides on biochemical and haematological parameters in Tunisian agricultural workers. **Journal of Exposure Science and Environmental Epidemiology**, Tunisia, v. 22, n. 3, p. 243-247, 2012.

ARAÚJO, A. J. Smoking treatment can impact COPD. **Pulmão RJ - Atualizacões Temáticas**, Rio de Janeiro, v. 1, n. 1, 2009.

ARAUJO, A. J.; LIMA, J. S.; MOREIRA, J.; JACOB, S. C.; SOARES, M. O.; MONTEIRO, M. C. M.; AMARAL, A. M.; KUBOTA, A.; MEYER, A.; COSENZA, C. A. N.; NEVES, C.MARKOWITZ, S. Multiple exposure to pesticides and health effects: cross-sectional study in a sample of 102 rural workers, Nova Friburgo, RJ. **Ciênc. Saúde Coletiva**, Rio de Janeiro, vol.12, n.1, p. 115-130, 2007.

ARCURY, T. A.; QUANDT, S. A.; CRAVEY, A. J.; ELMORE, R. C.; RUSSELL, G. B. Farmworker Reports of Pesticide Safety and Sanitation in the Work Environment. **American Journal of Industrial Medicine**, USA, v. 39, n. 5, p. 487-498, 2001.

ASPERLIN, A. Pesticide industry sales and usage-1992 and 1993 market estimates. **Environmental Protection Agency**, United States, p. 1-34, 1994.

AZEVEDO, M. F. A. Initial approach in outpatient care for neurotoxicological disorders. Part II - pesticides. **Revista Brasileira de Neurologia**, Rio de Janeiro, v. 46, n. 4, p. 21-28, 2010.

AZEVEDO, F. A.; CHASIN, A. A. M. **As Básicas Toxicológicas da Ecotoxicologia.** São Carlos: RIMA, 2003.

BALDI, I.; PIERRE, L.; MOHAMMED-BRAHIM, B.; LETENNEUR, L.; DARTIGUES, J. F.; BROCHARD, P. Neurodegenerative Diseases and Exposure to Pesticides in the Elderly. **Am J Epidemiol**, Oxford, v. 157, n. 5, p. 409-414, 2003.

BANERJEE, B. D.; SETH, V.; BHATTACHARYA, A.; PASHA, S. T.; CHAKRABORTY, A. K. Biochemical effects of some pesticide on lipid peroxidation and free-radical scavengers. **Toxicology Letters**, India, v. 107, p. 33-47, 1999.

BARTH, V. G.; BIAZON, A. C. B. Complications resulting from organophosphate poisoning. **SaBios: Rev. Saúde e Biol.**, Paraná, v. 5, n. 2, p. 2733, 2010.

BATISTA, E. S.; SABARENSE, C. M.; PRIORE, S. E.; ROSA, D. D.; MONTEZANO, I. M.; PELUZIO, M. C. G. Dietary habits, blood lipid levels and antioxidant status of young adult smokers and non-smokers. **Rev. Nutr.**, Campinas, v. 22, n. 3, p. 377-388, 2009.

BEDOR, C. N. G.; RAMOS, L.; PEREIRA, P. J.; REGO, M. A. V.; PAVÃO A. C.; AUGUSTO L. G. S. Vulnerabilities and risk situations related to the use of pesticides in irrigated fruit growing. **Rev. Bras. Epidemiol**, São Paulo, p. 39-49, 2009.

Evaluation and reflexes of the commercialisation and use of agrochemicals in the sub-middle region of the São Francisco valley. **Rev. Baiana Saúde Pública**, Bahia, p. 68-76. 2007.

BEDOR, C. N. G. **Study of the carcinogenic potential of pesticides used in fruit growing and its implications for health surveillance.**
Thesis (Doctorate in Public Health) - Oswaldo Cruz Foundation, Aggeu Magalhães Research Centre, Recife, 2008.

BELL, G. H.; DAVIDSON, J. N.; EMSLIE-SMITH, D. The formed elements of the blood. In: BELL, G. H.; DAVIDSON, J. N.; EMSLIE-SMITH, D. **Text book of physiology and biochemistry.** Churchill Livingstone: Edinburg, 1972.

BERLIN, A.; YODAIKEN, W. J.; LOGAN, D. C. International Seminar on the Assesment of Toxic Agents at the Workplace: roles of ambient and biological monitoring. **Int. Arch. Environm. Health**, USA, p. 197-207, 1982.

BERTAZZI, P. A.; ALESSIO, L.; DUCA, P. G. **Monitoraggio biologico negli**

ambienti di lavoro. Milano: Franco Angeli, 1988.

BHATT, M. H.; ELIAS, D. M. A.; MANKODI, A. K. Acute and reversible parkinsonism due to organophosphate pesticide intoxication: five cases. **Neurology**, Mumbai, v. 52, n. 7, p. 1467-1471, 2003.

BILA, D. M.; DEZOTTI, M. Endocrine disruptors in the environment: effects and consequences. **Chem. Nova,** Rio de Janeiro, v. 30, n. 3, p. 651-66, 2007.

BOCHNER, R. Sistema Nacional de Informações Tóxico-Farmacológicas - SINITOX and human poisoning by pesticides in Brazil. **Ciência e Saúde Coletiva**, Rio de Janeiro, v. 12, n. 1, p. 73-89, 2007.

BONASSI, S.; NERI, M.; PUNTONI, R. Validation of biomarkers as early predictors of disease. **Mutation Research**, Genova, p. 480-481,2001.

BRADY, N. C. **Nature and properties of soils.** 7. ed. Rio de Janeiro: Freitas Bastos, 1989.

BRAZIL. Ministry of Health. Department of Specialised Care. **Clinical protocols and therapeutic guidelines**. Brasília, DF, 2010.

BRAZIL. Ministry of Health. **FIOCRUZ SINITOX**. Available at: <http://www.fiocruz.br/sinitox_novo/cgi/cgilua.exe/sys/start.htm?tpl=home> Accessed on: 20 September 2011.

BRAZIL. Ministry of Health. Health Surveillance Secretariat. **Manual for the Surveillance of Populations Exposed to Pesticides.** Brasília: Pan American Health Organisation, 1997.

BOMHARD, E.; LOSER, E.; SCHILDE, B.(1981), [E605- Methyl] (Methyl parathion) chronic toxicological studies in rats (2 year feeding trial) Wuppartal - Elberfeld Bayer AG, Institute of toxicology IPCS -145, 155.

BRAZIL. Ministry of Health. Health Surveillance Secretariat. **Environmental health surveillance:** epidemiology texts. Brasília, DF, 2004.

BRAZIL. Ministry of Labour. Ordinance No. 24 of 29/12/94. Secretariat of Labour Safety. **Diario Oficial da União**, Brasília, DF, 30 December 1994.

BROWN, R.; LOCKWOOD, A.; SONAWANE, B. Neurodegenerative diseases: an overview of environmental risk factors. **Environ Health Perspect**, USA, v.113, n. 9, p. 1250-1256, 2005.

BRUNTON, L. L.; CHABNER, B. A.; KNOLLMANN, B. C.; GOODMAN, L. S. **Goodman & Gilman's the Pharmacological Basis of Therapeutics.** 12 ed. New

York: McGraw-Hill Professional, 2010.

BULL, D.; HATHAWAY, D. **Pragas e Venenos - Agrotóxicos no Brasil e no Terceiro Mundo.** 1. ed. Rio de Janeiro: Vozes, 1986.

BYDLOWSKI, S. P.; DE MOURA-NETO, R. S.; SOARES, R. P.; SILVA, R.; DEBES-BRAVO, A. A.; MORGANTI, L.. Genetic data on 12 STRs (F13A01, F13B, FESFPS, LPL, CSF1PO, TPOX, TH01, vWA, D16S539, D7S820, D13S317, D5S818) from four ethnic groups of São Paulo, Brazil. Forensic Sci Int. 2003 Jul 29;135(1):67-71.

CABELLO, G.; VALENZUELA, M.; VILAXA, A.; DURAN, V.; RUDOLPH, I.; HREPIC, N.; CALAF, G. A rat mammary tumour model induced by the organophosphorous pesticides parathion and malathion, possibly through acetylcholinesterase inhibition. **Environmental Health Perspectives**, Research Triangle Park, v. 109, n. 5, p. 471-479, 2001.

CALVERT, G. M.; PLATE, D. K.; DAS, R; ROSALES, R.; SHAFEY, O.; THOMSEN C.; MALE D.; BECKMAN, J.; ARVIZU, E.; LACKOVIC, M. Acute Occupational Pesticide-Related Illness in the US, 1998-1999: Surveillance Findings From the SENSOR-Pesticides Programme. **American Journal Of Industrial Medicine,** USA, p. 14-23, 2004.

CAMARGO, T. M.; ROCHA-JUNIOR, D. S.; FERREIRA, S. R.; VASCONCELOS, E. M. A.; OLIVEIRA, S. J.; SHITARA, E. S.; OSHIMA- FRANCO, Y. Influence of smoking on routine laboratory analyses: a pilot study in young adults. **Rev. Ciênc. Farm. Básica Apl.**, São Paulo, v. 27, n. 3, p. 247-251, 2006.

CASIDA, J. E.; NOMURA, D. K.; VOSE, S. C.; FUJIOKA, K. Organophosphate-Sensitive Lipases Modulate Brain Lysophospholipids, Ether Lipids and Endocannabinoids. **Chem Biol Interact**, Limerick, v. 175, n. 1-3, p. 355-364, 2008.

CAVALCANTE, T.; PINTO, M. **Considerations on tobacco and poverty in Brazil: Tobacco consumption and production.** Available at: <http://www.inca.gov.br/tabagismo/publicacoes/tabaco_pobreza.pdf>. Accessed on: 31 July 2011.

CARNEIRO, G.; RIBEIRO FILHO, F. F.; TOGEIRO, S. M.; TUFIK, S.; ZANELLA, M. T. 2007. Interactions between obstructive sleep apnoea syndrome and insulin resistance. **Arquivos Brasileiros de Endocrinologia e Metabologia**, São Paulo, v. 51, n. 7, p. 1035-1040, 2007.

CARVALHO, A. E.; SANTOS, I. G.; CURY, V. F. The influence of smoking on peridontal disease: Literature review. **SOTAU Revista Virtual de odontologia,**

Taubaté, v. 2, n. 5, p. 7 - 12, 2008.

CARVALHO, F. M.; NETO, A. M. S.; MENDES, J. L. B.; COTRIM' H. P.; NASCIMENTO'A. L. C.; JÚNIOR'A. S. L.; CUNHA, T. O. B. Alterations in Liver Enzymes in Oil Refinery Workers. **Rev. Saúde Pública**, São Paulo, v. 40, n. 1, p.92-8, 2006.

CHAIM, A. **History of spraying.** Available at: <http://www.agencia.cnptia.embrapa.br/recursos/Chaim_historialD-DcdtrOCVWI.pdf>. Accessed on: 21 October 2009.

CLAPP, R. W.; JACOBS, M. M.; LOECHLER, E. L. Environmental and Occupational Causes of Cancer New Evidence, 2005-2007. **Rev Environ Health**, Boston, v. 2, n. 1, p. 1-37, 2008.

COLOSSO, C.; TIRAMANI, M.; MARONI, M. Neurobehavioral effects of pesticides: state of the art. **Neurotoxicology**, Milan, p. 577-591, 2003.

COOPER, J.; DOBSON, H. The benefits of pesticides to mankind and the environment. **Crop Prot.**, UK, p. 1337-1348, 2007.

COSTA, J. A. C.; NETO, M. M.; NETO, O. M. V. Acute renal failure in intensive care. **Symposium: intensive care medicine: ii. selected topics**, Ribeirão Preto, p. 532-551, 1998.

COSTA, L. G.; COLE, T. B.; VITALONE, A.; FURLONG, C. E. Measurement of paraoxonase (PON 1) status as a potential biomarker of susceptibility to organophosphate toxicity. **Cilinal Chimica Acta**, Washington, v. 352, p. 3747, 2005.

COTRAN, R. S.; KUMAR, V.; ROBBINS, C. T. **Pathologia Estrutural e Funcional.** 6. ed. Rio de Janeiro: Guanabara Koogan S.A, 2000.

DAMS, R. I. Pesticides: Uses and dangers to health and the environment. **Saúde e Ambiente/Health and Environment Journal**, Balneário Camboriú, v. 7, n. 2, p. 37-44, 2006.

DELGADO, I. F.; PAUMGARTTEN, F. J. R. Poisoning and use of pesticides by farmers in the municipality of Paty do Alferes, Rio de Janeiro, Brazil. **Cad. Saúde Pública,** Rio de Janeiro, v. 20, n.1, p. 180-186, 2004.

DEPARTMENT OF RURAL SOCIOECONOMIC STUDIES. Tobacco growing and the framework convention: challenges for diversification, Curitiba-PR, 2009.

DRESSEL, T. D.; GOODALE, R. L.; ARNESON, M. A.; BORNER, J.W. Pancreatitis as a Complication of Anticholinesterase Insecticide Intoxication. **Annals Surgery**, Minnesota, v. 189, n. 2, p. 199-204, 1979.

DUFOUR D. R.; LOTT, J. A.; NOLTE, F. S.; GRETCH, D. R.; KOFF, R. S.; SEEFF, L. B. Diagnosis and monitoring of hepatic injury. I. Performance characteristics of laboratory tests. **Clin Chem,,** New York, v. 46, n. 12, p. 2027-2049, 2000.

ECOBICHON, D. J. Toxic effects of pesticides. In: KLAASSEN, C. D. **Casarett & Doll's toxicology**: the basic science of poisons. New York: McGraw-Hill, 2001.

ELLERY, A. E. L.; ARREGI, M. M. U.; RIGOTTO, R. M. Incidence of cancer in farmers in a cancer hospital in Ceará. In: XVIII World Congress of Epidemiology and VII Brazilian Congress of Epidemiology, 2008, Porto Alegre. **Proceedings...** Porto Alegre, 2008.

EL- SHAFEY, A. A. M.; SELIEM, M. M. E.; EL-MAHROUKY, F.; GABR, W. M.; KANDIL, R. A. Some Physiological and Biochemical Effects of Oshar Extract and Abamectin Biocide on Male Albino Rats. **Journal of American Science**, New York, v. 7, n. 12, p. 254, 261, 2011.

FAO - Food and agriculture organisation. **The world agricultural production**. Available at http://faostat.fao.org/site/339/default.aspx. Accessed: August 2009.

FAREEDA, M.; PATHAKA, M. K.; BIHARIA, V.; MUDIAMB, M. K. R.; PATELB, D. K.; MATHURA, N.; KUDDUSC, M.; KESAVACHANDRANA, C. N. Hematological and biochemical alterations in sprayers occupationally exposed to mixture of pesticides at a mango plantation in Lucknow, India. **Toxicological & Environmental Chemistry**, India, v. 92, n. 10, p. 19191928, 2010.

FARIA, N. M. X.; FASSA, A. G.; FACCHINI' L. A. Pesticide poisoning in Brazil: official information systems and challenges for epidemiological studies. **Ciênc. saúde coletiva**, Rio de Janeiro,v.12, n.1, 2007.

FARIA, N. M. X.; FACCHINI, L. A.; FASSA, A. G.; TOMASI, E. Rural production process and health in the Serra Gaúcha: a descriptive study. **Cad. Saúde Pública**, Rio de Janeiro, v. 16, n. 1, 2000.

. A cross-sectional study on the mental health of farmers in Serra Gaúcha (Brazil). **Rev. Saúde Pública**, São Paulo, v. 33, n. 4, p. 391-400, 1999.

FARIA, N.M.X.; FASSA, A. G.; FACCHINI, L.A. Pesticide poisoning in Brazil: official information systems and challenges for epidemiological studies. **Ciência & Saúde Coletiva**, Rio de Janeiro, v.12, n. 1, p. 25-38, 2007.

FARIA, N. M. X.; ROSA, J. A. R.; FACCHINI, L. A. Pesticide poisoning among rural fruit workers, Bento Gonçalves, RS. **Rev. Saúde Pública**, Rio de Janeiro, v. 43, n. 2, p. 335-344.

FARMER, P. B.; SINGH, R.; KAUR, B.; SRAM, R. J.; BINKOVA, B.; KALINA, I.; POPOV, T. A.; GARTE, S.; TAIOLI, E.; GABELOVA, A.; CEBULSKA-WASILEWSKA, A. Molecular epidemiology studies of carcinogenic environmental pollutants effects of polycyclic aromatic hydrocarbons (PAHs) in environmental pollution on exogenous and oxidative DNA damage. **Ocean & Coastal Management**, Leicester, p. 397-402, 2003.

FEDOSSI, O. A. **Organophosphate:** General Aspects and Analytical Methodology. 1991. Monograph (Specialisation in Social Toxicology) - UFF, Rio de Janeiro, 1991.

FEHLBERG, L. C.C.; LUTZ, L.V.; MOREIRA, A. H. Pesticides and their socio-cultural effects: Rural area of Valão de São Lourenço, Santa Teresa, ES, Brazil. **Natureza online**, Santa Tereza, v. 1, n. 2, p. 51-55. Available at:

http://naturezaonline.com.br/natureza/conteudo/pdf/Revista Online Fehlberg .pdf. Accessed on: 12 May 2012.

FERREIRA, H. S. Pesticides in Brazil: environmental impact and possible consequences of their interaction with human malnutrition. **Revista Brasileira de Saúde Ocupacional**, São Paulo, v. 80, n. 21, p. 51-60, 1999.

FILLA, G.; VESTENA, L. R.. Perception of the risk of poisoning due to the use of pesticides in Irati/PR. UNICENTRO - Revista Eletrônica Lato Sensu Ed.4 Year: 2008. ISSN: 1980-6116. Available at: http://web03.unicentro.br/especializacao/Revista Pos/P%C3%A1ginas/4%20 Edi%C3%A7%C3%A3o/Humanas/PDF/11-Ed4 CH-Percepc.pdf. Accessed on: May 2012.

FORGET, G. Pesticide and the third world. **J. Toxicol. Environ.** Canada, v. 32, n. 1, 11-31, 1991.

BRAZILIAN INSTITUTE OF GEOGRAPHY AND STATISTICS FOUNDATION. **2000 demographic census:** general characteristics of the population. Sample results. Available at: <http://www.ibge.gov.br>. 2000. Accessed on: 22 October 2009.

BRAZILIAN INSTITUTE OF GEOGRAPHY AND STATISTICS - IBGE. **2010 demographic census:** general characteristics of the population. Rio de Janeiro, 2010. Available at: <http://www.ibge.gov.br/estadosat/temas.php?sigla=al&tema=sis_2010>. Accessed on: 22 May 2012.

GARCIA, E. G. **Segurança e saúde no trabalho rural:** a questão dos agrotóxicos. São Paulo: Fundacentro, 2001.

GARCIA, E. G.; ALMEIDA, W. F. Exposure of rural workers to pesticides in Brazil. **Revista Brasileira de Saúde Ocupacional**, São Paulo, v. 19, n. 72, p. 7 - 11, 1991.

GONÇALVES, C. S.; GOMES, M. P. Z.; GONÇALVES, P. L.; GONÇALVES, L. L.; PEREIRA, F. E. L. Alcoholic Hepatitis. **J. bras. gastroenterol.**, Rio de Janeiro, v. 6, n. 2, p.59-68, 2006.

GUEDES, D. P.; GUEDES, J. E. R. P.; BARBOSA, D. S.; OLIVEIRA, J. A.. Tobacco use and plasma lipid-lipoprotein profile in adolescents. **Rev Assoc Med Bras**, São Paulo, v. 53, n. 1, p. 59-63, 2007.

GROOPMAN, J. D.; KENSLER, T. W. The light at the end of the tunnel for chemical-specific biomarkers: daylight or headlight? **Carciogenesis**, Baltimore, p.1-11, 1999.

HE, F.; CHEN, S.; TANG, X.; GAN, W.; TAO, B.; WEN. B. Biological monitoring of combined exposure to organophosphorus and pyrethroids. **Toxicol Lett**, China, p. 119-24, 2002.

HERNÁNDEZ A. F.; GÓMEZ, M. A.; PÉREZ, V.; GARCÍA-LARIO J. V.; PENA, G.; GIL, F; LOPEZ, O.; RODRIGO, L.; PINO, G.; PLA, A. Influence of exposure to pesticides on serum components and enzyme activities of cytotoxicity among intensive agriculture farmers. **Environ Res**, New York, p. 70-76, 2006.

HERNADEZ, A. F.; LÓPEZ, O.; GIL, F.; RODRIGO, L.; PLA, A.. Biomonitoring of workers with chronic exposure to plaguicides. Importancia de las esteras sanguíneas. **La Mutua**, Madrid, p. 35-50, 2006.

HERNÁNDEZ, A. F.; LÓPEZ, O.; RODRIGO, L.; GIL, F.; PENA, G.; SERRANO, J. L.; PARRÓN, T.; ÁLVAREZ, J. C.; LORENTE, J. A.; PLA, A. Changes in erythrocyte enzymes in humans long-term exposed to pesticides influence of several markers of individual susceptibility. **Toxicology Letters**, Spain, v. 159, p. 13-21, 2005.

HERRERA, A. O. Environment, Technology and Global Impoverishment. In: IBAMA. University and Environment Seminar. **Basic Documents...** Brasília: IBAMA, 1990.

HOSHINO, A. C. H. **Study of ototoxicity in workers exposed to organophosphates.** 2006. Master's thesis - UFRJ - Rio de Janeiro, 2006.

IBGE - Brazilian Institute of Geography and Statistics. Characteristics Demographic

Centre 2010: General characteristics of the population.Sample results.Available at http://www.ibge.gov.br/home/ accessed on 26 June 2012.

JACOBSON, H.; OSTERGAARD, G.; LAM, H.R.; POULSEN, M.E.; FRANDSEN, H.; LADEFOGED, O.; MEYER, O. Repeated dose 28-day oral toxicity study in Wistar rats with a mixture of five pesticides often found as residue in food: alphacypermethrin, bromopropylate, carbendazim, chlorpyrifos and mancozeb. **Food. Chem. Toxicol.**, Denmark, v. 42, n. 8, p. 1269-1277, 2004.

JAMAL, G. A. Long-term neurotoxic effects of organophosphate compounds. **Adverse Drug Reactions Toxicological Reviews**, Glasgow, v. 14, n. 2, p. 85-99, 1995.

JAYE, M.; LYNCH, K. J.; KRAWIEC, J.; MARCHADIER, D.; MAUGEAIS, C.; DOAN, K.; SOUTH, V.; AMIN, D.; PERRONE, M.; RADER, D. J. A novel endothelial-derived lipase that modulates HDL metabolism. **Nat Genet**, USA, p. 424-428, 1999.

JENSEN , H. K.; KONRADSEN ,F.; J0RS, E.; PETERSEN, J.; DALSGAARD, A. Pesticide Use and Self-Reported Symptoms of Acute Pesticide Poisoning among Aquatic Farmers in Phnom Penh, Cambodia. **Journal of Toxicology**. Washington, p. 1-8, 2011.

JOUSILAHTI, P.; RASTENYTE, D.; TUOMILEHTO, J. Serum gamma- glutamyl transferase, self-reported alcohol drinking, and the risk of stroke. **Stroke**, Dallas, p. 1851-1855, 2000.

JUNIOR , A. J. A.; COLBURN, W. A.; DEGRUTTOLA, V. G.; DEMETS, D. L.; DOWNING, G. J.; HOTH, D. F.; OATES, J. A.; PECK, C. C.; SCHOOLEY, R. T.; SPILKER, B. A.; WOODCOCK, J.; ZEGER, S. L. Biomarkers and surrogate endpoints: preferred definitions and conceptual framework. **Clin. Pharmacol. Therap.**, USA, v. 69, n. 3, p. 89-95, 2001.

JÚNIOR, J. F.; ALVES, M. E.; GUERREIRO, A.S. Organophosphate poisoning. **Medicina Interna**, Lisbon, v. 6, n. 2, 1999.

KAMEL, F.; HOPPIN, J. Association of pesticide exposure with neurologic dysfunction and disease. **Environ Health Perspect**, USA, v.112, n. 9, p.950- 958, 2004.

KAZMI, F.; SHAKOORI, A.R.; HAFEEZ, M.A.; ALI, S.S. Short-term effects of chlorpyrifos on haematology and biochemical components of blood of the Sprague-Dawley rats. **Pak. J. Zool.**, Pakistan, v. 35, n. 3, p. 245-257, 2003.

KHAN, D.A.; BHATTI, M.M.; KHAN, F.A.; NAQVI, S.T.; KARAM, A. Adverse Effects of Pesticides Residues on Biochemical Markers in Pakistani Tobacco Farmers. **International Journal of Clinical and Experimental Medicine**, New York , p. 274-282, 2008.

KLAASSEN, C. D. Non-metallic environmental toxicants: Air pollutants, solvents, vapours and pesticides. In: GOODMAN & GILMAN. **The pharmacological basis of therapeutics**. 8. ed. Rio de Janeiro: Guanabara Koogan, 1991.

KOH, D.; JEYARATNAM, J. Pesticides hazards in developing countries. **Sci Total Environ**, Amsterdam, p. 78-85, 1996.

KONRADSEN, F.; HOEK W. V. D.; COLE D. C.; HUTCHINSON G.; DAISLEY H.; SINGH S.; EDDLESTON, M. Reducing acute poisoning in developing countries: options for restricting the availability of pesticides. **Toxicology**, Copenhagen, v. 192, p. 249-261, 2003.

KUMMER, R.; SITTERT, N. J. V. Field studies on health effects from the application of two OP insectidide formulation by handheld ULV to cotton. **Toxicol. Lett.**, v. 33, p. 7-24, 1986.

KURT, P. H.; HOLMES, J. H. Changes Following Anticholinesterase Exposures - Blood Coagulation Studies. **Archives of Environmental Health**, Washington, p. 82-91, 1961.

LAM, P. K. S.; GREY, J. S. Predicting effects of toxic chemicals in the marine environment. **Marine Pollution Bulletin**, Hong Kong, p. 169-173, 2001.

LATORRACA, A.; MARQUES, G. J. G.; SOUSA, K. V.; FORNÉS, N. S. Pesticides used in tomato production in Goiânia and Goianápolis and effects on human health. **Com. Ciências Saúde**, Brasília, v. 19, n. 4, p. 365-374, 2008.

LEE, W. J.; HOPPIN, J. A.; BLAIR, A.; LUBIN, J. H.; DOSEMECI, M.; SANDLER, D. P.; ALAVANJA, M. C. R. Cancer incidence among pesticide applicators exposed to Alachlor in the Agricultural Health Study. **Am J Epid**, Rockville, v. 159, n. 4, p. 373-80, 2004.

LIMA, E. S.; COUTO, R. D. Structure, metabolism and physiological functions of high-density lipoprotein. **J. Bras. Patol. Med. Lab.**, Rio de Janeiro, v. 42, n. 3, p. 169-178, 2006.

LIMA, F.J. C.; MARQUES, P.R.B. O.; NUNES, G. S.; TANAKA, S. M. C. N. Organophosphate insecticide methamidophos: toxicological and analytical aspects. **Revista Ecotoxicologia e Meio Ambiente**, Curitiba, p. 17-34, 2001.

LONDON, F. . Pesticides in Brazil: a guide to action in defence of life. - Rio de

Janeiro: AS-PTA - Consultancy and Services for Alternative Agriculture Projects, 2011.
190 p. ISBN 978-85-87116-15-4. Available at: http://br.boell.org/downloads/Agrotoxicos-no-Brasil-mobile.pdf. Accessed on; 02 April 2012.

LONDON, L.; NELL, V.; THOMPSON, M. L.; MYERS, J. E. Effects of longterm organophosphate exposures on neurological symptoms, vibration sense and tremor among South African farm workers. **Scand J Work Environ Health**, South Africa, v. 24, p. 18-29, 1998.

MA, K.; CILINGIROGLU, M.; OTVOS, J. D.; BALLANTYNE, C. M.; MARIAN, A. J.; CHAN, L. Endothelial lipase is a major genetic determinant for high density lipoprotein concentration, structure, and metabolism, Houston. **PNAS**, v. 100, n. 5, 2003.

MACAN, J.; VARNAI V. M.; TURK, R. Health effects of pyrethrins and pyrethroids. **Arh Hig Rada Toksikol**, Zagreb, v. 52, n. 2, p. 237-243, 2006.

MACÁRIO, E. M. **Complexity and risks in the use of pesticides in agriculture: new questions for old issues.** 2001. 123f.
Dissertation (Master's) - Aggeu Magalhães Research Centre, Oswaldo Cruz Foundation, Recife, 2001.

MACHADO, J. M. H. Process of surveillance in workers' health. **Cadernos de Saúde Pública**, Rio de Janeiro, p. 33-46, 1997.

MARQUES, A. C. P. R.; CAMPANA, A.; GIGLIOTTI, A. P.; LOURENÇO, M. T. C.; FERREIRA, M. P.; LARANJEIRA, R. Consensus on the Treatment of Nicotine Dependence. **Revista Brasileira de Psiquiatria**, São Paulo, v. 23, n. 4, p. 200-214, 2001.

MARQUES, R. B. **Study of the epidemiological profile and evaluation of the treatment offered to patients with acute organophosphate insecticide poisoning treated at the Ceará Toxicological Assistance Centre (CEATOX) between February and July 2004, 2005.** 2005. Dissertation (Master's in Pharmaceutical Sciences) - Federal University of Ceará, Ceará, 2005.

MATSUDA K.; BUCKINGHAM, S. D.; KLEIER, D.; RAUH, J. J.; GRAUSO, M.; SATTELLE, D. B. Neonicotinoids: insecticides acting on insect nicotinic acetylcholine receptors. **Trends Pharmacol Sci**, Japan, v. 22, p. 573-580, 2001.

MATSUSHITA, T., MATSUI, Y., MATSUI, Y. Estimating mutagenic compounds generated during photolysis of fenitrotjion - by HPLC fractionation followed by mutagenicity testing and high-resolution GC-MS analysis. **Chemosphere**, Oxford, v. 64, n. 1, p. 144-155, 2005.

MATSUSHITA, T.; MATSUI, Y.; SAEKI, R.; INOUE, T. Mutagenicity of anaerobic fenitrothion metabolites after aerobic biodegradation. **Chemosphere**, Oxford, v. 61, p.1134-1141,2005.

MECDAD, A. A.; AHMED, M. H.; ELHALWAGY, M. E. A.; AFIFY, M. M. M. A study on oxidative stress biomarkers and immunomodulatory effects of pesticides in pesticide-sprayers. **Egyptian Journal of Forensic Sciences**, Cairo, p. 93-98, 2011.

MESQUITA, A. S.; OLIVEIRA, J. M. C. Tobacco growing in Bahia from excellence to decadence. **Bahia Agrícola**, Bahia, v. 6, n. 1, p. 31-40, 2003.

MEYER, A. CHRISMANA, J,; MOREIRA, J. C.; KOIFMAN, S. C. Cancer mortality among agricultural workers from Serrana Region, state of Rio de Janeiro, Brazil. **Environ Res**, Rio de Janeiro, v. 93, p. 264-271,2003.

MILHAM, S. Using multiple cause of death coding in occupational mortality studies. **Am J Ind Me**, Olympia, v. 14, n. 3, p. 341-344, 1988.

MILLER, G. T.; **Living in the Environment.** 12. ed., Wadsworth/Thomson Learning: Belmont, 2002.

MISRA, A.; KAPOOR, S.; MALHOTRA, O. P. Disseminated intarvascular coagulation caused by the insecticide Propoxur. **Postgraduate Medical Journal**, Oxford, p. 311-312, 1987.

MIYAMOTO, J.; KANEKO, H.; TSUJI, R.; OKUNO, Y. Pyrethroids, nerve poisons: how their risks to human health should be assessed. **Toxicology Letters**, Amsterdam, p. 933-40, 1995.

MOHAMMED, K. B.; MA, T. H. Tradescantia-micronucleus and -stamen hair mutation assays on genotoxicity of the gaseous and liquid forms of pesticides. **Mutation Research**, Amsterdam, p. 193-199, 1999.

MONTEIRO, C. **Acidity Theory in Atherosclerosis:** New Evidence. 1 ed. São Paulo, 2011.

MORAES, A. C. L. **Contribution to the study of carbamate poisoning: the case of chumbinho in Rio de Janeiro**. 1999. 111f. Master's Thesis - Oswaldo Cruz Foundation, National School of Public Health, Rio de Janeiro, 1999.

MOREIRA, J. C.; JACOB, S. C.; PERES, F.; LIMA. J. S.; MEYER, A.; OLIVEIRA-

SILVA, J. J.; SARCINELLI, P. N.; BATISTA, D. F.; EGLER, M.; FARIA, M. V. C.; ARAÚJO, A. J.; KUBOTA, A. H.SOARES, M. O.; ALVES, S. R.; MOURA, C. M.; CURI, R. Integrated assessment of the impact of pesticide use on human health in an agricultural community in Nova Friburgo, RJ. **Ciência & Saúde Coletiva**, Rio de Janeiro, v. 7, n. 2, p. 299 - 311,2002.
MORGAN, D. P. **Organophosphate**. 1998. Master's Thesis - International Healthcare Series, Colorado, United States of America, 1998.

MOURAD T. A. Adverse impact of insecticides on the health of Palestinian farm workers in the Gaza Strip: a haematologic biomarker study. **Int J Occup Environ Health**, Crete, v. 11, n. 2, p. 144-149, 2005.

NARAHASHI, T. Neuronal ion channels as the target sites of insecticides. **Pharmacology and Toxicology**, Copenhagen,p. 1-14, 1996.

NASUTI, C.; CANTALAMESSA, F.; FALCIONI, G.; GABBIANELLI, R. Different effects of type I and type II pyrethroids on erytrocyte plasma membrane properties and enzymatic activity in rats. **Toxicology**, Amsterdam, v. 191, n. 2, p. 233-244, 2003.

NEWCOMBE, D. Immune Surveillanee, Organophosphorus Exposure, and Lymmphomagenesis. **The Lancet**, London, p. 539-541, 1992.

NUNEZ, C. S.; BAILARTE, L. N.; SERRANO, M. C. M.; GONZÁLEZ, R. M. P. Biochemical-clinical study in people occupationally exposed to the action of agrochemicals and effects of their frequent use on health.
Ciencia e Investigación, San Marcos, v. 1, n. 1, 1998.

OERKE, E.C.; DEHNE, H. W. Safeguarding production-losses in major crops and the role of crop protection. **Crop Prot.**, Germany, v. 23, n. 4, p. 275-285, 2004.

OGA, S. **Fundamentos de Toxicologia.** 2. ed. São Paulo: Atheneu, 2003.

OLIVEIRA, P. H.; CATTANEO, R.; BORTOLOTTO, J. W. Evaluation of occupational health in rural workers exposed to pesticides in the north-west of the state of RS. In: XVI Mostra de iniciação científica, 2011, Rio Grande do Sul. **Proceedings**... Cruz Alta: UNICRUZ, 2011. Available at: <www.unicruz.edu.br/seminário>. Accessed on: 30 October 2011.

OLIVEIRA-SILVA, J. J.; ALVES, S. R.; MEYER, A.; PERES, F.; SARCINELLI, P. N.; MATTOS, R. C. O. C.; MOREIRA, J. C. Influence of socioeconomic factors on pesticide contamination, Brazil. **Revista de Saúde Pública**, São Paulo, v. 35, n. 2, p. 130-135, 2001.

OLIVEIRA-SILVA, J. J.; CASTRO, H. A; TRAMBELLINI, A. Search for new inflammatory biomarkers. In: CONGRESSO BRASILEIRO DE EPIDEMIOLOGIA, 5., 2002, Curitiba. **Proceedings**... Curitiba: 2002.

OLSSON, A. R.; SKOGH, T.; AXELSON, O.; WINGREN, G.. Occupations and exposures in the work environment as determinants for rheumatoid arthritis. **Occup Environ Med**, v. 61, n.3, p. 233-238, 2004.

INTERNATIONAL LABOUR ORGANISATION. Agriculture and natural resource-based sectors. Encyclopaedia of occupational health and safety, 3 ed., p. 64, 2001.

PARRÓN, T.; HERNANDEZ, A.F.; PLA, A.; VILLANUEVA, E. Clinical and Biochemical Changes in Greenhouse Sprayers Chronically Exposed to Pesticides. **Human and Experimental Toxicology**, Basingstoke, p. 957-963, 1996.

PATIL, J. A.; PATIL, A. J.; GOVINDWAR, S. P. Biochemical effects of various pesticides on sprayers of grape gardens. **Indian Journal of Clinical Biochemistry**, Kolhapur, v. 18, n. 2, p. 16-22, 2003.

PELAEZ, V. **Monitoring the Agrotoxics Market.** Available at: http://portal.anvisa.gov.br/wps/wcm/connect/c4bdf280474591ae99b1dd3fbc4c6735/study_monitoring.pdf?MOD=AJPERES. Accessed on: 09 August 2011.

PERES, F. J.; MOREIRA, C.; DUBOIS, G. S. Pesticides, health and the environment: an introduction to the subject. In: Peres, F.; Moreira, J. C. **Is it Poison or Medicine? - Agrotoxics, health and the environment**, Rio de Janeiro: FIOCRUZ, 2003.

PERES, F.; OLIVEIRA-SILVA, J. J.; DELLA-ROSA, H. V.; LUCCA, S. Challenges to the study of human and environmental contamination by pesticides. **Ciências & Saúde Coletiva**, Rio de Janeiro, v. 10, p. 27-37, 2005.

PIMENTEL, D. Green revolution agriculture and Chemical hazards. **Science of the total environment**, Netherlands, v.188, n. 1, p. 86-98, set. 1996.

PINHEIRO, N. L. **Evaluation of organophosphate poisoning in rural workers growing tomatoes (Lycopersicum esculentum Mill.) in the Caratinga region, MG**. 2008. Dissertation (Post-graduation in Environment and Sustainability) - Caratinga University Centre, Minas Gerais, 2008.

PINHEIRO, S.; SIVA, L. R.; CARVALHO, L. A.; FALK, J. W. Suicide and Illness Mental illness in Venâncio Aires - RS: a consequence of the use of organophosphate pesticides? **Preliminary research report**, Rio Grande do Sul, 1996.

PINHO, G. P.; NEVES, A. A.; QUEIROZ, M. E. L. R.. Analysing pesticide residues in tomatoes using matrix dispersion in solid phase (DMFS) and gas chromatography. **Quím. Nova,** São Paulo, v.32, n.1, p. 92-98, 2009.

PIRES, D. X.; CALDAS, E. D.; RECENA, M. C. P. Poisonings caused by agricultural pesticides in the micro-region of Dourados, Mato Grosso do Sul, Brazil, from 1992 to 2002. **Cadernos de Saúde Pública**, São Paulo, v. 21, n. 3, p. 804-814, 2005.

PIVETTA, F.; MACHADO, J. M. H.; ARAÚJO, U. C.; MOREIRA, M. F. R.; APOSTOLI, P. Biological monitoring: concepts and applications in public health. **Cad. Saúde Pública**, Rio de Janeiro, v.17, n.3, p. 545-554, 2001.

POSSAS, C. A.; TRAPÉ, A. Z. Saúde e trabalho no Campo: Da Questão Agrária à Política Previdenciária. **Cadernos do Internato Rural,** v. 2, n. 1, p. 13-19, 1983.

PRATT D. S.; KAPLAN, M. M. Laboratory Tests. In: SCHIFF E. R.; SORELL, M. F.; MADDREY, W. C. **Diseases of the Liver**. 8 ed. Philadelphia: Lippincott, 1999.

PRIGOL, M.; MARMENTINI, F.; GRAZZIOTIN, N. A.; MACEDO S. M. D. Effect of smoking on the lipid profile and its implications in inmates of the State Prison of Erechim-RS. **Rev. Bras. Anal. Clin.**, Rio de Janeiro, v. 39, n.1, p. 3-8, 2007.

QUANDT, S. A.; DORAN, A. M.; RAO, P.; HOPPIN, J. A.; SNIVELY, B. M.; ARCURY, T. A. Reporting Pesticide Assessment Results to Farmworker Families: Development, Implementation, and Evaluation of a Risk Communication Strategy. **Environmental Health Perspectives**. USA, v.112 , n.5, 2004.

QUIRENZE J. R. C. **Effect of ischaemic preconditioning on the early and intermediate phases of hepatic ischaemia and reperfusion injury in rats.** 2002. PhD Thesis - Federal University of São Paulo, Paulista School of Medicine, São Paulo, 2002.

RASTOGI S. K.; SINGH V. K.; KESAVACHANDRAN C.; JYOTI; SIDDIQUI M.; MATHUR N.; BHARTI R. S. Monitoring of plasma butyrylcholinesterase activity and haematological parameters in pesticide sprayers. **Indian J Occup Environ Med**, India, p. 29-32, 2008.

RASTOGI, S. K.; TRIPATHI, S; RAVISHANKER, D. A study of neurologic symptoms on exposure to organophosphate pesticides in the children of agricultural workers. **Indian J Occup Environ Med,** India, v. 14, n. 2, p. 5457, 2010.

RAY, G. **Pollution and Health.** New Delhi: Wiley Eastern Ltd., 1992.

RAY, D. E.; RICHARDS, P. G.. The Potential for Toxic Effects of Chronic, Low-Dose Exposure to Organophosphate. **Toxicol Lett**, Amsterdam, p. 343451,2001.

RECENA, M.C. P.; CALDAS, E. P.; PIRES, D. X.; PONTES, E. R. J. C. Pesticide exposure in Culturama, Brazil - Knowledge, attitudes, and practices. **Environmental Research**, Campo Grande, v. 102, n. 2, p. 230236, 2006.

REHNER, T. A.; KOLBO, J. R.; TRUMP R. ; SMITH, C. ; REID, D. Depression among victims of south Mississippi's methyl parathion disaster. **Health Soc Work**, USA, v. 25, p. 3-40, 2000.

ROBINSON, D.; WHITEHEAD, T. P. Effect of body mass and other factors on serum liver enzyme levels in men attending for well population screening. **Ann Clin Biochem** , London, p. 393-400, 1989.

ROCHA, M. O. C.; PEDROSO, E. R. P.; FONSECA, J. G.; SILVA, O. A. **Terapêutica Clínica.** 2. ed. Rio de Janeiro: Guanabara Koogan S.A., 1998.

ROTHLEIN, J.; ROHLMAN, D.; LASAREV, M.; PHILLIPS, J. MUNIZ, J.; MCCAULEY, L. Organophosphate pesticide exposure and neurobehavioral performance in agricultural and nonagricultural Hispanic workers. **Environ Health Perspect**, USA, v.114, n. 5, p.691-696, 2006.

RITZ, B.; YU, F. Parkinson's disease mortality and pesticide exposure in California 1984-1994. **Int J Epidemiol**, Los Angeles, v. 29, p. 323-329, 2000.

RUIZ, A. **Toxicidad crónica por plaguicidas en trabajadores de invernadero de la zona básica de salud de Níjar (Almería).** 1997. Thesis (Doctorate) - University of Granada, Granada, 1997.

SAADEH, A. M.; ALALY, M. K.; FARSAKH, N. A.; GHANI, M. A. Clinical and socio demographic future of acute carbamate and organophosphate poisoning: a study of adult patients in North Jordan. **Journal of toxicology - Clinical toxicology**, New York, v. 34, p. 45-51, 1996.

SALVI, R.M.; LARA, D.R.; GHISOLFI, E.S.; PORTELA, L.V.; DIAS, R.D.; SOUZA, D.O. Neuropsychiatric Evaluation in Subjects Chronically Exposed to Organophosphate Pesticides. **Toxicol Sci**, Oxford, v. 72, n. 2, p. 267-71, 2003.

SANTOS, N.S.J.; DRAIBE, S. A.; KAMIMURA, M. A.; CUPPARI, L. Serum albumin as a nutritional marker for haemodialysis patients. **Rev. Nutr.**, Campinas, v.17, n. 3, p.339-349, 2004.

SANTOS, V. M. R.; DONNICI C. L.; COSTA, J. B. N.; CAIXEIRO, J. M. R. Pentavalent organophosphorus compounds: history, synthetic methods of preparation and applications as insecticides and antitumour agents. **Quim Nova**, v. 30, n. 1, p.159-70, 2007.

SCHAUMBURG H. H.; BERGER, A. R. Human toxic neuropathy due to industrial agents. In: DYCK, P. J.; THOMAS, P. K. (Org.) **Peripheral Neuropathy**. London:

Saunders, 1993. p. 1533-1548.

SHARMA, R.; CHISTI, Y.; BANERJEE, U. C. Production, Purification, Characterisation and Application of Lipases. **Biotechnology Advances**, India, p. 627-662, 2001.

SCHERER, G. Biomonitoring of inhaled complex mixtures - Ambient air, diesel exhaust and cigarette smoke. **Experimental And Toxicologic Pathology**, Muenchen, p. 75-110, 2005.

SCHOENHALS, M.; FOLLADOR, F. A. C.; SILVA, C. Analysing the environmental impacts of tobacco farming on the health of tobacco farmers and environmental management initiatives in the tobacco industry. **Engenharia Ambiental - Espírito Santo do Pinhal**, v. 6, n. 2, p. 16-37, 2009.

SEFRINI, G. **Tobacco in Brazil and the world.** 1. ed. Santa Cruz do Sul: AFUBRA, 1995.

SELANDER S.; CRAMER K. Interrelationships between lead in blood, lead in urine, and ALA in urine during lead work. **British Journal of Industrial Medicine**, Gothenburg, p. 28-39, 1970.

SALEEM, M. A.; AHMAD, M.; ASLAM, M.; SAYYED, A. H. . Resistance to selected organochlorin, organophosphate, carbamate and pyrethroid, in Spodoptera litura (Lepidoptera: Noctuidae) from Pakistan. Pakistan. **J Econ Entomol.** 2008 Oct;101(5):1667-75.PMID:18950050[PubMed - indexed for MEDLINE]

SENANAYAKE, N.; PEIRES, H. Mortality due to poisoning in a developing agricultural country: trends over 20 years. **Human and experimental toxicology,** Basingstoke, v. 14, p. 808-11, 1995.

SCHILDE, B. & BOMHARD, E. (1984) (E 605-methyl (Methyl parathion) supplementary histopathological test further to the 2 year feeding trials on rats Addendum to report No. 9889.Wuppertal-Elberfeld, Bayer A. G. Ins. of toxicology. (unpublished report No. 12559 submitted to WHO by Bayer AG. Leverkusen Germany).

SHUGART, L. R. DNA damage as a biomarker of exposure. **Ecotoxicology**, Oak Ridge, p. 329-340, 2000.

SILVA, C. M. S., FAY, E. F. Characteristics of the soil environment. In: SILVA, C.M.S.; FAY, E. F. **Agrotoxics and the environment.** Brasília: Embrapa, 2004.

SILVA, J. M. **Process of work and conditions of exposure to pesticides: the case of vegetable growers in Baldim, Minas Gerais, Brazil.** Master's thesis - Federal University of Minas Gerais, Belo Horizonte, 2000.

SILVA, J. M.; NOVATO-SILVA, E; FARIA, H. P.; PINHEIRO, T. M. M. Agrotoxico e trabalho: uma combinação perigosa para a saúde do trabalhador rural. **Ciênc. saúde coletiva**, Belo Horizonte, v. 10, n. 4, p. 891903, 2005.

SILVA, R. C. L.; MARQUES, M. Women diagnosed with acute myocardial infarction, implications for nursing care practice in coronary units. **Rev. Meio Amb. Saúde**, Minas Gerais, v. 2, n.1 p.195-242, 2007.

SIQUEIRA, S. L.; KRUSE, M. H. L. Agrotoxics and human health: the contribution of health professionals. **Revista da Escola de Enfermagem USP**, São Paulo, v. 42, n. 3, p. 584-590, 2008.

SMIT, A. M.; WENDEL, V.; JOODE, B. N.; HEEDERIK, D.; PEIRIS-JOHN, R. J.; HOEK, W. V. D. Neurologic symptoms among Sri Lankan farmers occupationally exposed to acetylcholinesterase- inhibiting insecticides. **Am J Ind Med**, Colombo, v. 44, p. 254-264, 2003.

SOARES, L. F. **Acute Carbamate** Poisoning **in Paediatrics. Epidemiological, Clinical and Therapeutic Aspects.** 1998. Monograph (Specialisation in Paediatrics) - UFF, Rio de Janeiro, 1998.

SOARES W.; ALMEIDA R. M. V. R.; MORO, S. Rural labour and risk factors associated with pesticide use in Minas Gerais, Brazil. **Cadernos de Saúde Pública,** Rio de Janeiro, v. 19, n.4, 2003.

SOARES, W. L.; FREITAS, E. A. V.; COUTINHO, J. A. G. Rural labour and health: pesticide poisoning in the municipality of Teresópolis - RJ. **Rev. *Econ. Sociol. Rural*,** Rio de Janeiro, v. 43, n. 4, p. 685-701,2005.

SODERLUND, D. M.; CLARK, J. M.; SHEETS, L. P.; MULLIN, L. S.; PICCIRILLO, V. J.; SARGENT, D.; STEVENS, J. T.; WEINER, M. L. Mechanisms of Pyrethroid Neurotoxicity: implications for cumulative risk assessment. **Toxicology**, Amsterdam, 2001.

SODRE, F. L.; COSTA, J. C. B.; LIMA, J. C. C. Evaluation of renal function and injury: a laboratory challenge. **J. Bras. Patol. Med. Lab.**, Rio de Janeiro, v. 43, n. 5, p. 329-337, 2007.

SOTH, T.; HOSOKAWA, M. Organophosphate and their impacts on the global environment. **Neurotoxicology**, Amsterdam, p. 1-4, 2000.

SOUZA, A. A. R. M.; SOUZA, A. C.; WINK, M.; SIQUEIRA, I. R.; FERREIRA, M. B. C.; FERNANDES, L.; HIDALGO, M. P. L.; TORRES, I. L. S. Evaluation of the impact of exposure to pesticides on the health of the rural population: Vale do Taquari (RS, Brazil). **Ciênc. saúde coletiva**, Rio de Janeiro, v.16, n. 8, p. 3519-

3528, 2011.

SPADOTTO, C. A.; GOMES, M. A. F; LUCHINI, L. C.; ANDRÉA, M. M. **Monitoring the Environmental Risk of Pesticides: principles and recommendations.** Available at: <http://www.cnpma.embrapa.br/public/conta.php3?flag=54>. Accessed on: 11 January 2011.

STALLONES, L. Suicide Mortality Among Kentucky Farmers, 1979-1985. **Suicide Life Threat Behav**, New York, v.20, n. 2, p. 156-63, 1990.

STALLONES, L.; BESELER, C. Pesticide Poisoning and Depressive Symptoms Among Farm Residents. **Ann. Epidemiol**, New York, v. 12, n. 6, p. 389-94, 2002.

STALLONES, L.; LEFF, M.; GARRET, C.; CRISWELL, L.; GILLAN, T. Depressive Symptoms Among Colorado Farmers. **NASD Rev**, p. 1-5, 1995.

STOPELLI, M. B. S.; MAGALHÃES, C. P. Segurança e saúde alimentar: a questão dos agrotóxicos. **Journal Ciência & Saúde Coletiva**, Rio de Janeiro, p. 91-100, 2005.

TERRY, A.V. J. Functional consequences of repeated organophosphate exposure: Potential non-cholinergic mechanisms.**Pharmacol Ther,** Oxford, v. 134, n. 3, p. 355-65, 2012.

TERRY, A.V.; STONE, J. D.; BUCCAFUSCO, J. J.; SICKLES, D. W.; SOOD, A.; PRENDERGAST, M. A. Repeated Exposures to Subthreshold Doses of Chlorpyrifos in Rats: Hippocampal Damage, Impaired Axonal Transport, and Deficits in Spatial Learning. **J. Pharmacol. Exp. Ther.**, v. 305, n. 1, p. 375384, 2003.

TOMIZAWA, M.; CASIDA, J. E. Selective toxicity of neonicotinoids attributable to specificity of insect and mammalian nicotinic receptors. **Annu. Rev. Entomol**, Berkeley, v. 48, p. 339-364, 2003.

. Neonicotinoid insecticide toxicology: Mechanisms of selective action. **Annu. Rev. Pharmacol. Toxicol.**, Berkeley, v. 45, p. 247-268, 2005.

TRAPÉ, A. Z. The case of pesticides. In: ROCHA, L. E.; RIGOTTO, R. M.; BUSCHINELLI, J. T. P. **Is this people's work? Life, illness and work in Brazil**, Petrópolis: Editora Vozes, 1994.

TSATSAKIS, A.M.; ZAFIROPOULOS, A.; TZATZARAKIS, M.N.; TZANAKAKIS, G.N. & KAFATOS A.Relation of PON1 and CYP1A1 Genetic Polymorphisms to Clinical Findings in a Cross-Sectional Study of a Greek Rural

Population Professionally Exposed to Pesticides. **Toxicology Letters**, Amsterdam, v. 186, p. 66-72, 2009.

VAINIO, H. Biomarkers in the identification of risks, especially with regard to susceptible persons and subgroups. **Scand J Work Environ Health**, Stockholm, p. 1-3, 1999.

VALE, N. B.; DELFINO, J. Anaesthesia in the black population. **Rev. Bras. Anestesiol.**, Campinas, v.53, n. 3, p. 401-418, 2003.

VASCONCELOS, T. H. C.; MODESTO-FILHO, J.; DINIZ, M. F. F. M.; SANTOS, H. B.; AGUIAR, F. B.; MOREIRA, P. V. L. Acute preclinical toxicological study with the hydroalcoholic extract of the leaves of Cissus sicyoides L. (Vitaceae). **Rev. bras. Farmacogn**, João Pessoa, v.17, n.4, 2007.

VERGER, R. "'Interfacial Activation of Lipases': Facts or Artifacts", **Trends in Biotechnology,** France, p. 32-38, 1997.

VICENTE, M. C. M. BAPTISTELLA, C. S. L.; COELHO, P. J.; JÚNIOR, A. L. Perfil do aplicador de agrotóxicos na agricultura paulista. **Informações Econômicas**, São Paulo, v. 28, n.11, 1998.

WALKER H.K.; HALL, W. D.; HURST, J. W. **CLINICAL METHODS:** The History, Physical, and Laboratory Examinations. 3 ed. Boston: Butterworths,1990.

WANNAMETHEE, G.; EBRAHIM, S.; SHAPER, A. G. Gamma-glutamyltransferase: determinants and association with mortality from

ischemic heart disease and all causes. **Am J Epidemiol**, Oxford, p. 699708, 1995.

WARD, J. B.; HENDERSON, R. E. Identification of Needs in Biomarker Research. **Environmental Health Perspectives**, Mexico, v. 104, n. 5, p. 895-900, 1996.

WEIZMAN, Z.; SOFER, S. Acute Pancreatitis in Children With Anticholinesterase Insecticide Intoxication. **Pediatrics**, Evanston, v. 90, n. 2, p. 204-206, 1992.

WHITEHEAD, T. P.; ROBINSON, D.; ALLAWAY, S. L. The effects of cigarette smoking and alcohol consumption on serum liver enzyme activities: a dose-related study in men. **Ann Clin Biochem**, London, p. 530-535, 1996.

WHO. 1989. Environmental Health Criteria 93: Chlorophenols other than pentachlorophenol. World Health Organisation. Geneva, 207 pp.

ZIEMEN, M. Thrombozytenfunktion und Plasmatische Gerinnung nach Intoxikation mit Organophosphaten. **Klinische Wochenschrift**, Berlin, p. 814-820, 1984.

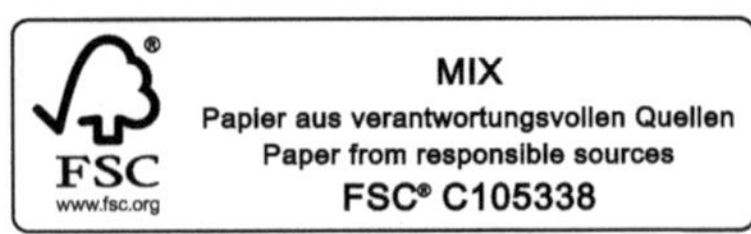

Printed by Books on Demand GmbH, Norderstedt / Germany